# The Art and Science of Emergency Nursing: A Professional Guide

Carl A. Killian, RN, BSN, CEN

**Copyright © 2024 Carl A. Killian**

All rights reserved. No part of this book may be reproduced, stored in a retrieval system, or transmitted in any form or by any means, electronic, mechanical, photocopying, recording, or otherwise, without prior written permission of the publisher, except for the inclusion of brief quotations in a review.

## Acknowledgements

I would like to express my deepest gratitude to all those who have contributed to the development and completion of The Art and Science of Emergency Nursing: A Professional Guide. To my colleagues at Johns Hopkins Hospital, thank you for your unwavering support and for fostering an environment that continually inspires excellence in emergency nursing. I am particularly grateful to my mentors who have guided me throughout my career and helped shape my understanding of the critical role emergency nurses play in patient care.

A heartfelt thanks to my family and friends for their encouragement and patience during the writing process. Lastly, I would like to acknowledge the countless emergency nurses around the world whose dedication and commitment to patient care inspire me every day. This book is a tribute to your work and the impact you make in the lives of patients and their families.

## Preface

Emergency nursing is a dynamic and demanding field that sits at the intersection of science, art, and human compassion. It requires a unique blend of technical expertise, clinical judgment, and the ability to adapt to high-pressure situations while delivering exceptional patient care. The Art and Science of Emergency Nursing: A Professional Guide was conceived as a comprehensive resource to empower current and aspiring emergency nurses to excel in their practice, deepen their understanding of critical concepts, and embrace the multidisciplinary nature of this specialty.

As healthcare systems evolve, emergency departments have become pivotal access points for individuals across the spectrum of acute and chronic illnesses. Emergency nurses, as frontline professionals, are tasked with managing diverse patient populations—from trauma victims to patients with complex medical conditions. This book serves as both a foundational text and a practical reference, addressing the core principles of emergency nursing while exploring advanced techniques, critical care interventions, and evidence-based practices.

Drawing from years of professional experience and collaboration with leaders in emergency medicine, The Art and Science of Emergency Nursing is designed to bridge theory and practice. It provides clear explanations of clinical procedures, strategies for prioritizing care, and insights into the psychosocial aspects of emergency nursing. Key features of this guide include:

1. Comprehensive Coverage: Chapters span a wide array of topics, including triage protocols, trauma management, pediatric emergencies, geriatric considerations, and the integration of technology in emergency care.

2. Evidence-Based Practice: Content is grounded in the latest research, ensuring that readers are equipped with up-to-date knowledge and techniques.

3. Case Studies and Clinical Scenarios: Real-world examples highlight common challenges encountered in emergency nursing and provide strategies for effective decision-making.

4. Professional Development: Practical advice is offered to help nurses navigate career progression, certification, and leadership roles within emergency care settings.

5. Holistic Approach: The book emphasizes the importance of cultural competence, communication skills, and interdisciplinary collaboration in delivering patient-centered care.

This book is not just a technical manual but a testament to the resilience, dedication, and critical thinking that define the profession of emergency nursing. It is written for a diverse audience, including novice nurses entering the field, seasoned practitioners seeking to refine their skills, educators developing curricula, and administrators aiming to improve departmental efficiency and patient outcomes.

I hope that this guide inspires readers to approach emergency nursing with curiosity, confidence, and a commitment to excellence. Whether you are responding to a mass casualty incident, supporting a patient during a mental health crisis, or managing routine yet critical interventions, your work is invaluable.

It is my honor to contribute to the professional growth of emergency nurses worldwide. Together, we continue to advance the art and science of this vital discipline.

**Carl A. Killian, RN, BSN, CEN**
Emergency Nursing Specialist
2024

**Acknowledgement**
**Preface**
**Table of Contents**
**List of Abbreviations**


### Table of contents

## Chapter 1
Emergency Nursing: An Evolving Profession

- Overview of Emergency Nursing
- Historical Development and Advancements
- The Future of Emergency Nursing

## Chapter 2
The Emergency Nurse as a Professional

- Core Competencies and Skills
- Professionalism in Practice
- Ethical Considerations in Emergency Care

**Chapter 3**
Types of Emergency Departments

- Levels of Emergency Care
- Structure and Function of Various Emergency Departments
- Organizational Roles in Emergency Settings

**Chapter 4**
The Role of the Emergency Nurse in Triage

- The Triage Process
- Triage Systems and Protocols
- Decision-Making and Prioritization in Triage

**Chapter 5**
Risk Management and Quality Issues in Emergency Nursing

- Identifying and Addressing Risk Factors
- Patient Safety in the Emergency Department
- Continuous Quality Improvement Practices

**Chapter 6**
Challenging Patient Populations in the Emergency Department

- Care for Vulnerable and High-Risk Patients
- Managing Pediatric and Geriatric Populations
- Addressing Mental Health and Substance Abuse Issues

**Chapter 7**
The Emergency Nurse and the Abused Patient

- Recognizing Signs of Abuse
- Protocols for Caring for Abused Patients

- Legal and Ethical Responsibilities in Handling Abuse Cases

**List of Abbreviations**

ACLS – Advanced Cardiovascular Life Support

BSN – Bachelor of Science in Nursing

CEN – Certified Emergency Nurse

ED – Emergency Department

EMS – Emergency Medical Services

EMT – Emergency Medical Technician

HIPAA – Health Insurance Portability and Accountability Act

IV – Intravenous

JCAHO – Joint Commission on Accreditation of Healthcare Organizations

NREMT – National Registry of Emergency Medical Technicians

RN – Registered Nurse

SANE – Sexual Assault Nurse Examiner

TBI – Traumatic Brain Injury

# Chapter 1
# Emergency Nursing: An Evolving Profession

Defining Emergency Nursing

The American Nurses Association (ANA) defines nursing as the act of safeguarding, advancing, and optimizing health and abilities. It involves preventing illnesses and injuries, alleviating suffering through diagnosis and treatment, and advocating for individuals, families, and communities (ANA, 2015). An emergency, meanwhile, refers to a critical and unexpected situation requiring immediate care due to illness or injury. Emergency nursing, a specialized field within the profession, addresses these situations by delivering rapid, patient-centered care.

This chapter examined the history of emergency nursing, the role of the emergency department (ED), the foundational principles of emergency nursing, and the key components of this specialized practice.

## Historical Perspective on Emergency Nursing

In the past, healthcare was provided at the site of injury or illness, as hospitals and emergency departments did not exist. Emergency care traces its roots to wartime practices, particularly during the Middle Ages, when care evolved out of necessity. Monasteries or churches sometimes provided additional support, but systematic emergency care was lacking.

In modern history, the World Health Assembly's Resolution 60.22 in 2012 marked a significant step in global emergency care development, highlighting the importance of accessible systems worldwide (Anderson et al., 2012). However, disparities in emergency care systems persist, often highlighted during crises such as the Ebola outbreak (2014) and the Nepal earthquake (2015).

Florence Nightingale's Contributions to Emergency Nursing

Florence Nightingale is regarded as a pioneer of emergency nursing. During the Crimean War in 1854, she organized field nursing services, prioritizing care for the most critically ill or injured soldiers. Her contributions included implementing measures like reducing overcrowding, improving sanitation, and advocating for patient welfare.

Nightingale's work extended beyond emergency care; she founded the Nightingale Training School in 1865, advancing professional nursing education. Her advocacy for patients, particularly marginalized groups, set the foundation for the critical role of patient advocacy in emergency nursing today (Ayers, 2014).

Advances in the 20th Century

The 20th century saw significant developments in emergency nursing. Early initiatives, like the "First Aid Room" at the Henry Street Settlement under Lillian Wald, provided basic care to underserved populations. Nurses began operating under standing orders, a precursor to today's protocols (Snyder et al., 2006).

The demand for emergency services grew rapidly, with hospitals establishing emergency rooms to accommodate increasing patient needs. By the mid-20th century, emergency medicine and nursing emerged as distinct specialties, driven by wartime experiences and societal changes, including the evolving role of women. Nurses played a crucial role in triage and acute care during World War II, the Korean War, and the Vietnam War, underscoring their value in collaborative, multidisciplinary care.

The Birth of the Emergency Nurses Association (ENA)

The establishment of the Emergency Nurses Association (ENA) in 1970 marked a milestone for the profession. Founded by Anita Dorr and Judith Kelleher, the ENA unified emergency nursing and provided a platform for advocacy, education, and professional development. Over time, the organization has grown to represent over 40,000 members and continues to lead initiatives for evidence-based emergency care.

The ENA remains instrumental in shaping the profession through position statements, training programs, and publications, ensuring that emergency nurses are equipped to meet the evolving demands of their field.

Emergency Nurses Association (ENA) Educational Resources for Emergency Nursing

The key educational resources provided by the ENA, designed to enhance the knowledge and skills of emergency nurses at various stages of their careers are outlined below.

1. Trauma Nursing Core Course (TNCC)

Purpose: TNCC is an internationally recognized program that establishes a standardized knowledge base for trauma nursing.

Details:

A two-day course focusing on core trauma nursing knowledge and psychomotor skills.

Aims to refine practical skills and build a foundational understanding of trauma management.

2. Emergency Nursing Pediatric Course (ENPC)

Purpose: Designed to improve pediatric patient care by equipping nurses with essential knowledge and confidence.

Details:

A two-day program covering pediatric emergencies.

Enhances the ability to manage pediatric patients in emergency settings by focusing on core-level skills.

3. Course on Advanced Trauma Nursing (CATN)

Purpose: Provides advanced trauma education for experienced emergency nurses, emphasizing critical thinking and early complication management.

Details:

Online, self-paced learning with seven contact hours and six interactive modules.

Focus areas:

Advanced pathophysiology in trauma care.

Evidence-based strategies for long-term trauma management.

Designed for both individual and group study.

4. Geriatric Emergency Nursing Education (GENE)

Purpose: An e-learning program addressing the specific needs of older adults in emergency care.

Details:

Evidence-based curriculum for recognizing atypical presentations and improving geriatric outcomes.

Focuses on assessment tools, coordination of care, and specialized geriatric interventions.

Advanced Practice Nursing in Emergency Settings

The evolution of advanced practice roles in emergency nursing highlights significant historical milestones and ongoing developments.

Historical Background

1965: Pediatric Nurse Practitioner program launched at the University of Colorado to address underserved pediatric populations, setting the stage for advanced practice nursing.

1970s: Expansion of emergency nurse practitioner (ENP) roles through certificate programs lasting 16–68 weeks, emphasizing clinical skills like history-taking, physical examinations, and wound care.

1976: University of Virginia's ENP program introduced, requiring two years of nursing experience and ED physician mentorship, with optional master's degree opportunities.

Current Developments

Curriculum: Programs now include advanced resuscitation techniques, psychosocial counseling, and diagnostic evaluations.

ENA Guidelines: The 1999 Scope of Practice document formalized ENP roles, with subsequent competency studies enhancing emergency care standards.

Global Practice: ENPs have become integral to ED teams worldwide, particularly in underserved areas.

Role of the Emergency Department (ED)

Emergency departments serve as critical care points for diverse populations, from uninsured patients to those requiring urgent stabilization.

Challenges and Trends

Overcrowding: Rising ED visits (136+ million annually as of 2011) are compounded by staff shortages and limited inpatient capacities.

Triage Evolution: Nurses remain pivotal in triage, a method essential for prioritizing care amidst increasing patient volumes.

Legislation and Social Impact

EMTALA (1986): Mandates that all patients, regardless of citizenship or financial status, receive emergency care.

Affordable Care Act: Expanded insurance coverage led to increased ED usage, challenging resource allocation.

Public Perception: Media and television glamorizing emergency care contribute to public reliance on EDs for non-emergent issues.

Emergency Nursing as a Recognized Specialty

Definition and Scope

American Nurses Association (ANA): Emergency nursing was officially recognized in 2011, defined as short-term, episodic care for undiagnosed physical or emotional health issues.

ENA Guidelines: Emphasizes interventions ranging from minimal to life-saving and the importance of prevention and stabilization across diverse settings.

Professional Standards and Ethics

The ENA Code of Ethics underpins emergency nursing, advocating for:

Multidisciplinary collaboration.

Competence and accountability.

Patient advocacy and public health improvements.

## Just Culture

Promotes an environment where staff can report errors without fear, fostering transparency and safety improvements.

## Standards of Professional Performance

Key standards include education, evidence-based practice, communication, and ethical decision-making. These principles ensure high-quality care and support the evolving role of emergency nurses in complex care environments.

## Summary

Emergency nursing is a specialized field focused on providing care to individuals of all ages who present with acute or undiagnosed physical or emotional health conditions. This care is often episodic, primary, and short-term, delivered in various settings (American Nurses Association [ANA], 2011; Bonalumi & King, 2007; Fazio, 2010; Patrick, 2010).

Pioneering nurses Anita Dorr and Judith Kelleher were instrumental in establishing emergency nursing as a recognized specialty. Their efforts culminated in the creation of the Emergency Nurses Association, which continues to support and promote the field globally.

Emergency departments (EDs) manage a broad spectrum of cases, ranging from life-threatening conditions like cardiopulmonary arrest to minor ailments. Emergency nurses are indispensable to ED operations, requiring distinct competencies and extensive experience. As societal and healthcare challenges evolve, the practice of emergency nursing continues to adapt, ensuring it meets the complex needs of patients. These nurses remain central to delivering emergency care, embodying its core values and mission.

References

1. American College of Emergency Physicians (ACEP). (2014, May 21). ER visits up since implementation of the Affordable Care Act [news release]. Retrieved from http://newsroom.acep.org/2014-05-21-ER-Visits-Up-Since-Implementation-of-Affordable-Care-Act#Closed

2. American Nurses Association (ANA). (2011, August 23). ANA recognizes emergency nursing as a specialty [Press release]. Retrieved from http://www.nursingworld.org/FunctionalMenuCategories/MediaResources/PressReleases/2011-PR/ANA-Recognizes-Emergency-Nursing-Specialty-Practice.pdf

3. Bonalumi, N., & King, D. (2007). Professionalism and leadership. In S. Hoyt & J. Selfridge-Thomas (Eds.), Emergency nursing core curriculum (6th ed., pp. 1046–1056). Philadelphia, PA: W. B. Saunders.

4. Emergency Nurses Association (ENA). (2011). Emergency nursing scope and standards of practice. Des Plaines, IL: Emergency Nurses Association.

5. Fazio, J. (2010). Emergency nursing practice. In P. Kunz Howard & R. Steinmann (Eds.), Sheehy's emergency nursing: Principles and practice (6th ed., pp. 8–15). St. Louis, MO: Mosby Elsevier.

# Chapter 2
# The Emergency Nurse as a Professional

Understanding Professionalism in Nursing

Professionalism in nursing extends beyond merely demonstrating appropriate behaviors in clinical settings. It represents a continuous commitment to ethical principles, core personal values, and societal expectations, regardless of whether a nurse is on or off duty. This ethos is rooted in a nurse's moral code and is essential for maintaining public trust—a cornerstone of nursing licensure. Actions that compromise this trust, whether during professional or personal activities, may result in disciplinary measures, including license revocation.

While licensure serves as the baseline for professionalism, it represents only an entry-level standard. True professional growth involves advancing through self-improvement, accountability, advocacy, and meaningful contributions to the field. This journey is supported by mentorship, experiential learning, and scholarly endeavors. As Conard and Pape (2014) emphasize, professionalism requires nurses to engage in activities that foster teaching, research, and evidence-based practice.

Creating a Legacy Map

Rather than focusing solely on career achievements, nurses are encouraged to adopt a "legacy map" approach to identify long-term contributions to the profession. Hinds et al. (2015) define a legacy map as a personal plan for influencing healthcare by sharing knowledge and improving care outcomes. This concept encourages nurses to reflect on their aspirations and goals, asking:

What improvements in nursing can be attributed to my efforts?

How do I want to be remembered by my colleagues and patients?

What enduring impact do I aim to leave on the profession and beyond?

These introspections help professionals align their career paths with meaningful objectives that contribute to their sense of fulfillment and professional well-being.

Evidence-Based Practice: A Cornerstone of Modern Nursing

Historically, nursing practices were guided by tradition and physician directives rather than evidence. However, the past three decades have seen a paradigm shift toward incorporating scientific inquiry into routine care. Evidence-based practice (EBP) is now integral to nursing, encompassing empirical research, clinical expertise, and patient-centered care.

Despite this progress, obstacles remain. Yoder et al. (2014) identified barriers such as limited time, resources, and research knowledge among nurses, which hinder EBP implementation. Moreover, some nurses perceive evidence application as the responsibility of unit educators or specialists, rather than frontline staff. Addressing these challenges requires fostering a culture of inquiry and equipping nurses with the tools to critically appraise and apply research.

Clinical Practice Guidelines (CPGs)

Clinical practice guidelines provide evidence-based frameworks for standardized patient care. Emergency nurses play a crucial role in translating these guidelines into actionable bedside practices. High-quality CPGs are often derived from rigorously appraised evidence and are available through trusted sources like the National Guidelines Clearinghouse, the CDC, and professional organizations such as the Emergency Nurses Association (ENA).

By leveraging these resources, nurses can ensure that their interventions are supported by the strongest available evidence, optimizing patient outcomes and advancing the profession.

Engaging in Evidence-Based Literature

To keep pace with advancements in healthcare, nurses must approach their practice with an inquisitive mindset. Engaging in evidence-based literature reviews and fostering discussions within clinical teams are effective strategies for promoting EBP. Activities such as journal clubs and interprofessional collaborations encourage critical thinking and knowledge dissemination, ultimately enhancing patient care delivery.

Translating Research to Practice

The ultimate test of nursing competency lies in the ability to translate research findings into practical interventions. However, as Carman et al. (2013) caution, the applicability of research to specific clinical settings must be thoroughly evaluated. Differences in resources, policies, and culture can influence the success of evidence translation. Thus, careful adaptation and ongoing evaluation are crucial to ensure the successful integration of research into clinical practice.

Learning Opportunities for Emergency Nurses

Emergency nurses have access to a wide range of educational opportunities, both formal and informal, to enhance their professional skills and knowledge. These include hospital-based training programs, mandatory or elective in-service education, external conferences, and academic programs leading to degrees such as BSN, MSN, MBA, DNP, or PhD. Selecting the most suitable options depends on individual needs, available resources, and personal circumstances.

Modern Approaches to Nursing Education

Traditional lecture-based education has given way to innovative learning methods, such as hands-on and case-based instruction. Simulation labs in hospitals and nursing schools have gained prominence, offering realistic clinical scenarios to help nurses practice and refine essential skills. High-fidelity manikins and healthcare actors allow for immersive learning experiences, facilitating skill development in areas such as practical techniques and interpersonal communication.

Team-based simulations involving interdisciplinary professionals like physicians, nurses, and allied health staff foster collaboration and teamwork, promoting enhanced patient care.

Attending Conferences
Conferences provide valuable opportunities for professional growth. Events like the Emergency Nurses Association Annual Conference allow participants to learn about the latest advancements in emergency nursing while

networking with colleagues facing similar challenges. These gatherings can also facilitate the formation of long-term professional relationships.

International conferences offer a global perspective, showcasing how resource constraints are managed in different healthcare systems and fostering innovative problem-solving. Such cross-cultural exchanges encourage deeper professional connections and broaden perspectives on emergency nursing issues.

Funding Educational Pursuits

Limited institutional funding often necessitates personal financial investment for attending regional or national conferences. Strategies to mitigate costs include:

Establishing a savings plan to fund conference attendance every 1–3 years.

Deducting educational expenses as professional costs for tax purposes, adhering to IRS guidelines.

Leveraging loyalty programs for reduced travel and accommodation expenses.

Sharing costs, such as room-sharing with colleagues or seeking discounted rates.

Joining professional organizations offering discounts or scholarships for conference attendance.

Presenting posters or speaking at conferences can also reduce or waive registration fees and provide opportunities for skill enhancement in public speaking and publication.

Academic Advancement

Pursuing higher education is vital for career progression. Nurses with diploma or associate degrees are encouraged to complete a BSN, particularly as hospitals seek Magnet® designation, requiring 80% of nursing staff to hold baccalaureate degrees. Tuition assistance may be available for this purpose.

Higher academic degrees, such as MSN, DNP, or PhD, support advanced practice roles and academic aspirations. Strategic planning, maintaining high academic performance, and building professional relationships with faculty are key to seamless progression through academic programs.

Specialty Certification

Certification demonstrates professional excellence, validating a nurse's specialized knowledge and skills. It is often required for career advancement and may lead to higher pay or clinical ladder progression. Certifications also benefit healthcare institutions by meeting accreditation standards and improving patient outcomes.

Barriers and Strategies

Barriers to certification include test anxiety, costs, and lack of institutional support. Effective preparation strategies include:

Using study guides and sample questions.

Participating in review courses.

Forming study groups for peer support.

Some certifications, such as the Sexual Assault Nurse Examiner (SANE) or advanced practice certifications, require specific educational credentials or clinical experience. Maintaining multiple certifications demands significant effort and expense but reflects a high level of professional expertise.

Upholding Institutional Policies and Procedures

Emergency nurses bear a professional responsibility to understand and adhere to their workplace's institutional policies and procedures. These guidelines are designed to align with regulatory standards established by federal, state, and local authorities, as well as accrediting organizations like the Centers for Medicare & Medicaid Services (CMS), The Joint Commission, and the American College of Surgeons Committee on Trauma. They also reflect evidence-based practices and institution-specific protocols. Familiarity with these policies serves as a critical safeguard against professional liability, as outlined by Balestra (2012).

Failure to comply with institutional protocols can have significant repercussions, including personal, professional, and organizational liabilities, regulatory penalties, and employment sanctions. It is crucial to recognize that institutional policies cannot override federal or state laws. For instance, if state law prohibits nurses from delegating intravenous catheter insertion to unlicensed personnel, adherence to a conflicting hospital policy could result in charges of professional misconduct.

Given the extensive nature of institutional policies, memorizing all of them is unrealistic. Nurses must know where to access relevant guidelines and consult them as needed to ensure compliance. When policies are unclear or incomplete, leveraging the administrative chain of command for clarification is vital. Nurses can play a proactive role in identifying gaps in existing policies, advocating for updates based on current best practices, and contributing to the development of revised guidelines. These efforts provide opportunities for professional growth, leadership development, and the promotion of evidence-based practices.

In some cases, institutional policies may impede optimal care delivery or create unnecessary burdens. These policies must be revised through effective advocacy, supported by data and expert opinions. The complexity of the revision process depends on whether the policy is institutionally derived or tied to external regulations, with the latter requiring more time and resources. Advocacy for policy improvements is an essential aspect of professionalism, ensuring that institutional practices align with current standards and patient care needs.

Participating in Institutional Committees

Serving on institutional committees offers emergency nurses an invaluable avenue for professional growth and influence. Committees address system-wide issues, many of which intersect with emergency care. Nurses contribute critical insights to strategic planning and problem-solving, fostering a culture of shared responsibility. Berkow et al. (2012) emphasized that engaging frontline nurses in organizational goal-setting enhances their sense of ownership and commitment.

Committee involvement broadens nurses' perspectives, building connections across departments and providing insights into healthcare operations at institutional, community, and national levels. This exposure enriches understanding of organizational initiatives and facilitates effective communication with emergency department (ED) colleagues. As Needleman and Hassmiller (2009) observed, integrating frontline nurses into decision-making strengthens institutional systems and drives sustainable improvements.

Before joining a committee, nurses should thoroughly understand the group's mission, goals, and expectations. If participation requirements are unfeasible, it is prudent to decline the opportunity, ensuring representation by someone who can meet the demands. Common committee focuses include patient care access, quality and safety, infection prevention, nurse staffing, and electronic medical records.

Active and professional engagement is essential for committee success. Attendance, punctuality, and adherence to meeting protocols are critical. Respectful communication, attentiveness, and a balanced perspective enhance collaboration and support effective decision-making. Additionally, nurses should ensure ED leadership is involved when committee recommendations affect departmental operations.

Despite the added responsibilities, committee participation provides significant professional benefits. It fosters leadership skills, expands networks, and positions nurses for career advancement. Institutional initiatives also benefit from the contributions of engaged nursing staff, as frontline involvement is key to achieving quality outcomes. Needleman and Hassmiller (2009) highlighted the importance of embedding improvement efforts into daily practice, supported by active staff participation and adequate resources.

Joining Professional Organizations

Membership in professional nursing organizations demonstrates a commitment to the field beyond workplace expectations. As Guerrieri (2010) noted, these organizations serve as the public face of the nursing profession and provide members with valuable resources. Common benefits include forums for collaboration, continuing education opportunities, evidence-based practice guidelines, research funding, and political advocacy.

Additional perks often include access to professional journals, discounts on educational resources, liability insurance, and certification fees. Some organizations maintain repositories of institutional policies and templates, simplifying the development of such documents for members' facilities.

Joining a professional organization is typically straightforward, requiring an application and payment of dues. Some groups, however, have specific eligibility criteria and review processes. Membership offers opportunities to stay informed about advancements in the field, engage with peers, and access tools that enhance professional development.

Through active participation in professional organizations, nurses can contribute to the advancement of their specialty while gaining knowledge, networking opportunities, and resources to support their practice.

Advocacy and Legislative Influence in Emergency Nursing

Advocating for legislative and regulatory changes is a critical responsibility for emergency nurses, enabling them to expand their impact on healthcare at both professional and societal levels. A comprehensive understanding of the political system and the skills to act as a change agent are essential for initiating meaningful reforms. Legislative action often proves to be a powerful mechanism for driving lasting changes, especially when other approaches fall short. Whether focusing on enhancing patient care or improving nurses' working conditions, advocacy efforts can yield significant benefits for both healthcare providers and patients.

Effective advocacy requires the ability to influence others, a core professional competency. The American Nurses Association (ANA) Code of Ethics for Nurses defines advocacy as "the act or process of pleading for, supporting, or recommending a cause or course of action." This can encompass advocating for individuals, groups, or broader societal issues, such as global health initiatives. Moreover, the ANA emphasizes the duty of nurses to actively participate in policy-making by serving on institutional committees, engaging in civic activities, or taking on leadership roles in healthcare advocacy. Similarly, the Emergency Nurses Association (ENA) aligns its mission with advocating for patient safety and excellence in emergency nursing practice, further emphasizing the role of nurses in shaping healthcare policies.

Emergency nurses have demonstrated their influence in legislative processes by addressing critical issues such as workplace violence. For example, as of February 2013, 37 states enacted laws categorizing assaults on emergency nurses as misdemeanors or felonies, illustrating the profession's ability to drive public policy. Nurses have also supported legislative initiatives targeting public health concerns, including mandatory helmet laws and restrictions on smoking in public spaces. Statutory measures often achieve broader compliance and more significant societal impact than traditional health education efforts due to the enforceability of legal requirements.

Legislative advocacy begins with recognizing the need for change and deciding to act. This can range from contacting legislators through written or verbal communication to organizing collective efforts with other healthcare professionals. Advocacy efforts may involve presenting data, sharing personal stories, drafting regulatory proposals, and testifying at legislative hearings. Such activities may occur at various levels, from local governance to national policy-making, and offer opportunities for professional growth and improved patient outcomes.

For nurses new to political involvement, mentorship from experienced nurse advocates and formal education in health policy can provide valuable guidance. Many professional organizations offer resources, such as templates for legislative campaigns, internship programs, and opportunities to engage with policymakers. Establishing relationships with political figures or supporting their campaigns can further enhance advocacy efforts, creating networks that may facilitate future legislative actions. Some nurses may even pursue advanced degrees in health policy to deepen their expertise and leadership in this arena.

The Role of Volunteering in Professional Development

Volunteering reflects a commitment to service and embodies the core values of altruism and citizenship in emergency nursing. By contributing their expertise in various settings, emergency nurses can make meaningful contributions to society while gaining personal and professional fulfillment. Despite some perspectives that nursing efforts should always be financially compensated, volunteering offers invaluable experiences, including the development of skills in teaching, leadership, and clinical practice. These opportunities often lead to expanded networks, professional recognition, and enhanced career prospects.

Emergency nurses can volunteer in diverse roles, such as teaching cardiopulmonary resuscitation (CPR), participating in health screenings, or providing first aid at community events. Longer-term commitments may include serving as parish nurses, staffing clinics in underserved areas, or supporting local emergency medical services during rescue operations. For those interested in global health, humanitarian aid and disaster response missions offer opportunities to work in resource-limited environments and engage with diverse cultures. However, these roles require careful planning, including financial considerations, time commitments, and employer support.

By aligning their passions with available resources, nurses can find fulfilling volunteer opportunities without overextending themselves. Volunteering not only enriches personal growth but also contributes to the nursing profession's collective impact on health and wellness.

Personal Professional Liability Insurance in Emergency Nursing

The emergency department (ED) is a dynamic and often unpredictable environment, especially from a legal perspective. While most nurses are not typically named in lawsuits, emergency nurses frequently deliberate on whether to invest in personal professional liability insurance. Compared to the high premiums for physicians, the cost of liability insurance for registered nurses (RNs) is generally affordable, often under $200 annually. Advanced practice nurses (APNs), however, face higher premiums depending on their specialty and scope of practice.

In many cases, when employed by a healthcare system, nurses are covered under the facility's corporate liability policy for malpractice claims. Given this coverage, some nurses may perceive personal liability insurance as an unnecessary expense. However, several key factors make carrying personal liability insurance a wise consideration:

1. Professional Status 24/7: As a professional, your actions outside the employer relationship can result in claims that are not covered by the employer's insurance. For instance, offering

healthcare advice outside of your role may lead to personal liability.

2. Licensure Protection: Complaints filed with the professional licensing board about your conduct, whether from an employer or the public, may not be covered by the employer's liability policy. Personal insurance provides legal defense for licensure protection in these situations.

3. Post-Employment Claims: If you separate from your employer and a claim arises, the employer's liability policy may no longer cover defense costs. A personal policy would continue to provide protection even after employment ends.

In addition to covering malpractice, personal liability insurance often includes licensure protection and may offer benefits such as legal representation during a deposition, reimbursement for defense expenses, and access to educational resources. The cost of the policy may vary depending on state regulations and the insurer's assessment of malpractice risk.

It is important to note that personal liability policies generally do not cover criminal acts. Therefore, selecting a reputable insurance provider is crucial. Nurses are encouraged to choose insurers that offer:

Advisory boards for seeking solutions to professional issues.

License protection to defend against administrative or disciplinary actions.

Coverage for incidents at previous employers.

Sufficient coverage levels (e.g., $1 million/$3 million malpractice, $25,000 disciplinary coverage per occurrence).

The option to select an attorney for disciplinary defense.

Resources such as risk management educational materials and discounts for continuing education on these topics.

Health Promotion and Injury Prevention in Emergency Nursing

Emergency nurses are uniquely positioned to engage in injury prevention and health promotion, given their exposure to a wide range of patient conditions, from pediatric to geriatric care. Many of the injuries and illnesses seen in the ED could be preventable or less severe with better choices or behaviors. Thus, educating patients on health risks, lifestyle choices, and injury prevention is a key professional responsibility for emergency nurses.

The Emergency Nurses Association (ENA) Code of Ethics emphasizes the duty of emergency nurses to educate the public about healthy lifestyles, general well-being, and injury prevention. This includes delivering education not only in the clinical setting but also in the broader community.

While health promotion efforts are commonly part of discharge instructions, emergency nurses can also capitalize on the "teachable moment" during patient care in the ED. This approach allows for a more in-depth discussion on modifiable health risks. For instance, nurses might educate patients on how high-sodium diets exacerbate heart conditions or how poor blood glucose control impacts diabetes management.

One notable intervention is the Screening Brief Intervention and Referral to Treatment (SBIRT), which aims to identify and intervene with patients who have risky drinking behaviors. A study by Désy et al. (2010) demonstrated that SBIRT, when delivered by ED nurses, significantly reduced alcohol consumption by 70% in the intervention group, compared to 20% in the control group. Furthermore, the intervention group had fewer repeat ED visits

(20% vs. 31% in the usual care group). Despite its potential benefits, implementing SBIRT in the ED faces challenges such as ED overcrowding and staff resistance to new programs.

For pediatric emergency nurses, both the child and their family require attention in health education. Family habits, such as smoking or improper use of child safety seats, directly impact a child's health. Nurses can use these interactions as opportunities to educate families on the dangers of exposure to environmental tobacco smoke (ETS) and the importance of proper child passenger safety.

Additionally, ED nurses play a crucial role in helping patients navigate the healthcare system. Effective discharge teaching can help patients better manage their recovery and reduce the likelihood of needing to return to the ED. Gozdzialski et al. (2012) found that thorough discharge education enhances patient understanding of recovery expectations and the resources available for follow-up care.

While the ED is a key setting for health promotion, there are barriers to effective patient education. The fast-paced environment, staff limitations, and patient readiness to learn can hinder these efforts. However, creative strategies such as providing educational videos, printed materials, and follow-up phone calls can help overcome these obstacles and improve patient engagement in health promotion.

Community-Based Health Education

Participating in community-based education extends the reach of health promotion and injury prevention beyond individual patient encounters. These programs, which can be offered through schools, community organizations, and health agencies, provide nurses with the opportunity to educate a broader audience about health risks, disease prevention, and healthy lifestyle choices.

For example, nurses in coastal areas have developed community outreach programs like

"ED Beach Reach" to address marine-related injuries and drowning prevention. By providing educational materials and interacting directly with beachgoers, they were able to raise awareness and potentially reduce the incidence of these injuries.

These community programs are crucial in spreading important health messages, and their impact can be amplified when shared through professional networks, such as the Emergency Nurses Association (ENA). Pelton (2012) advocates for nurse involvement in such outreach, which aligns with the core values of emergency nursing professionalism.

In summary, emergency nurses play an essential role in promoting health, preventing injuries, and educating patients both within the ED and the community. While facing challenges in the fast-paced ED environment, the integration of health education into patient care can lead to better patient outcomes and a broader public health impact.

References

1. Agency for Healthcare Research and Quality (AHRQ). (n.d.). National guideline clearinghouse. Retrieved from www.guideline.gov

2. Altman, M. (2011). Let's get certified: Best practices for nurse leaders to support a culture of certification. AACN Advanced Critical Care, 22(1), 68–75.

3. American Nurses Association. (2015). Code of ethics for nurses with interpretive statements. Retrieved from http://www.nursingworld.org/MainMenuCategories/EthicsStandards/CodeofEthicsforNurses/Code-of-Ethics-For-Nurses.html

4. American Nurses Credentialing Center (ANCC). (2013, June 7). Magnet Recognition Program® FAQ: Data and expected outcomes. Retrieved from http://nursecredentialing.org/Magnet/MagnetFAQs/MagnetFAQCategory/MagnetFAQs/MagnetFAQ-OrganizationalOverview#007

5. Balestra, M. (2012). The best defense for registered nurses and nurse practitioners: Understanding the disciplinary process. Journal of Nursing Law, 15(2), 39–44. Retrieved from http://dx.doi.org/10.1891/1073-7472.15.2.39

6. Berkow, S., Workman, J., Aronson, S., Stewart, J., Virkstis, K., & Kahn, M. (2012). Strengthening frontline nurse investment in organizational goals. Journal of Nursing Administration, 42(3), 165–169.

7. Board of Certification for Emergency Nursing. (2015). BCEN spotlight. Retrieved from https://www.bcencertifications.org/Home.aspx

8. Bureau of Labor Statistics. (2015, February 25). Volunteering in the United States, 2014. Retrieved from http://www.bls.gov/news.release/volun.nr0.htm

9. Carman, M. J., Wolf, L. A., Baker, K. M., Clark, P. R., Henderson, D., Manton, A., & Zavotsky, K. E. (2013). Translating research to practice: Bringing emergency nursing research full circle to the bedside. Journal of Emergency Nursing, 39(6), 657–659. doi: http://dx.doi.org/10.1016/j.jen.2013.09.004

10. Carnegie, E., & Kiger, A. (2009). Being and doing politics: An outdated model or

21st century reality? Journal of Advanced Nursing, 65(9), 1976–1984. doi: 10.1111/j.1365-2648.2009.05084.x

11. Clutter, P. C. (2009). Clinical practice guidelines: Key resources to guide clinical decision making and enhance quality health care. Journal of Emergency Nursing, 35, 460–461.

12. Conard, P. L., & Pape, T. (2014). Roles and responsibilities of the nursing scholar. Pediatric Nursing, 40(2), 87–90.

13. Dawson, S., & Freed, P. E. (2008). Nurse leadership: Making the most of community service. The Journal of Continuing Education in Nursing, 39(6), 268–273.

14. Deckter, L., Mahabee-Gittens, M., & Gordon, J. S. (2009). Are pediatric ED nurses delivering tobacco cessation advice

to patients? Journal of Emergency Nursing, 35(5), 402–405.

15. Désy, P. M., Howard, P. K., Perhats, C., & Li, S. (2010). Alcohol screening, brief intervention, and referral to treatment conducted by emergency nurses: An impact evaluation. Journal of Emergency Nursing, 36(6), 538–545. doi: 10.1016/j.jen.2009.09.011

16. Emergency Nurses Association. (2013, February 25). Workplace violence penalties and terminology database. Retrieved from https://www.ena.org/government/State/Documents/WPVPenalties.pdf

17. Emergency Nurses Association (ENA). (2015a). Code of ethics. Retrieved from https://www.ena.org/about/Documents/CodeofEthics.pdf

18. Emergency Nurses Association (ENA). (2015b). Mission statement. Retrieved from https://www.ena.org/about/Pages/Default.aspx

19. Gozdzialski, A., Schlutow, M., & Pittiglio, L. (2012). Patient and family education in the emergency department: How nurses can help. Journal of Emergency Nursing, 38(3), 293–295. doi: http://dx.doi.org/10.1016/j.jen.2011.12.014

20. Guerrieri, R. (2010). Professional growth: Learn, grow and bloom by joining a professional association. Nursing 2010, 40(5), 47–48.

21. Harding, A. D., Walker-Cillo, G. E., Duke, A., Campos, G. J., & Stapleton, S. J. (2013). A framework for creating and evaluating competencies for emergency nurses. Journal of Emergency Nursing,

39(3), 252–264. doi: http://dx.doi.org/10.1016/j.jen.2012.05.006

22. Hearrell, C. L. (2011). Advocacy: Nurses making a difference. Journal of Emergency Nursing, 37, 73–7.

23. Hinds, P. S., Britton, D. R., Coleman, L., Engh, E., Humble, T. K., Keller, S., ... Walczak, D. (2015). Creating a career legacy map to assure meaningful work in nursing. Nursing Outlook, 63(2), 211–218.

24. Howard, P. K., & Papa, A. M. (2012). Future-of-nursing report: The impact on emergency nursing. Journal of Emergency Nursing, 38(6), 549–552. doi: 10.1016/j.jen.2012.08.001

25. Institute of Medicine (IOM). (2011). The future of nursing: Leading change,

advancing health. Washington, DC: The National Academies Press.

26. Internal Revenue Service (IRS). (2015, January 15). Tax benefits for education: Information center. Retrieved from http://www.irs.gov/uac/Tax-Benefits-for-Education:-Information-Center

27. Kaplow, R. (2011). The value of certification. AACN Advanced Critical Care, 22(1), 25–32.

28. Kendall-Gallagher, D., Aiken, L. H., Sloane, D. M., & Cimiotti, J. P. (2011). Nurse specialty certification, inpatient mortality, and failure to rescue. Journal of Nursing Scholarship, 43(2), 188–194. doi: 10.1111/j.1547-5069.2011.01391.x

29. Montgomery, T. M. (2012). Health care and politics: Making your voice heard. Nursing for Women's Health, 16(3),

198–201. doi: 10.1111/j.1751-486X.2012.01730.x

30. Needleman, J., & Hassmiller, S. (2009). The role of nurses in improving hospital quality and efficiency: Real-world results. Health Affairs, 28(4), w625–w633. Retrieved from http://content.healthaffairs.org/content/28/4/w625.full.html

# Chapter 3
# Types of Emergency Departments

Overview of Emergency Department (ED) Environments

Different emergency departments (EDs) vary significantly in their facilities, resources, and patient care approaches, shaped by factors such as hospital size, community needs, and the local healthcare market. These differences play a crucial role in defining the scope of services offered and can impact the healthcare professionals' career decisions. Recognizing the diversity among EDs helps healthcare providers choose an environment that aligns with their career aspirations and provides the most opportunities for professional growth.

Hospital Types and Their Impact on Emergency Care

Hospitals adopt various organizational structures that reflect their mission, financial model, and the community they serve. These structural choices influence the quality and scope of emergency services offered. In the United States, all hospitals with an ED must comply with the Emergency Medical Treatment and Labor Act (EMTALA). This law ensures that all patients presenting with an emergency, regardless of their financial situation, receive necessary care. However, EMTALA applies only to emergencies and does not extend to non-emergent or inpatient conditions.

In rural areas, hospitals are often more specialized in handling local types of trauma, such as agricultural accidents, while urban hospitals tend to see more penetrating trauma or accidents related to high-density environments. Even though both rural and urban hospitals provide emergency care for conditions like heart attacks, the availability of specialized services like interventional cardiology can differ significantly.

For-Profit Hospitals

For-profit hospitals operate similarly to other businesses, aiming to generate a profit by providing healthcare services. These hospitals may be publicly or privately owned, with the former trading stocks on public markets like the New York Stock Exchange. For-profit hospitals are motivated by the need to meet revenue expectations from investors while balancing patient care outcomes. Service expansions in such hospitals often target high-revenue areas, such as advanced imaging technologies. However, these hospitals also receive federal subsidies, known as "outlier payments," to cover cases with unusually high costs.

Non-Profit Hospitals

Non-profit hospitals, under Section 501 of the Internal Revenue Code, operate primarily to serve charitable, scientific, or public safety needs, making them exempt from property, sales, and income taxes. Though nonprofits can generate revenue, any surplus is reinvested in the hospital's operations and mission, which often includes community service. Larger non-profit systems may experience more financial resilience due to pooled resources and collaborative efforts with other hospitals.

Faith-Based Hospitals

Faith-based hospitals, often rooted in religious beliefs, are a subset of non-profit hospitals that focus on serving the community as part of a spiritual mission. For example, Catholic hospitals are responsible for a significant portion of inpatient care in the U.S. These hospitals often have specific ethical guidelines that influence healthcare delivery. For instance, faith-based hospitals may not provide certain procedures that conflict with their religious principles. Despite their non-profit status, faith-based hospitals face scrutiny, particularly when government funding intersects with religious values, as seen in debates about limiting certain medical services.

Teaching Hospitals

Teaching hospitals serve as key centers for medical education, research, and patient care. These hospitals offer cutting-edge treatment and participate in clinical trials that contribute to the development of new therapies. Medical students and residents receive hands-on training alongside established healthcare professionals, which can result in a higher number of care team members per patient. Teaching hospitals often have access to more specialized resources and handle complex cases that may not be common in other hospitals.

Critical Access Hospitals

Critical Access Hospitals (CAHs) are rural hospitals designated by the federal government to receive higher reimbursement rates from Medicare and Medicaid. To qualify as a CAH, the hospital must meet specific criteria, such as being located more than 35 miles from the nearest hospital and having no more than 25 inpatient beds. These facilities are essential in providing emergency services to remote areas, despite their limited size and resources. CAHs must maintain a 24-hour emergency service to meet the needs of their communities.

Veterans Affairs Facilities

Veterans Affairs (VA) facilities are specialized hospitals designed to meet the needs of military veterans. These government-run institutions are supported by federal funds and provide care tailored to the unique needs of veterans, such as treating combat-related injuries and mental health conditions. VA hospitals often participate in research, particularly in areas like prosthetics and trauma care, thanks to their involvement in military-specific care advancements.

Active Military Hospitals

Active military hospitals serve members of the armed forces and often lead the way in trauma care innovations. These facilities, ranging from battlefield units to more permanent military hospitals, play a key role in advancing emergency care, particularly in trauma resuscitation. The outcomes of trauma care in military settings are often exceptional, offering valuable insights into trauma treatment that have been adopted in civilian hospitals. Military hospitals are at the forefront of emergency care research, with a focus on improving survival rates in critical trauma cases.

Specialty Emergency Departments: Overview and Categorization

Emergency departments (EDs) in the United States are organized into various categories based on their services and capabilities. These categories can vary across states, reflecting differences in licensing requirements and the level of care provided.

1. Standby Emergency Department: In this setting, basic nursing services are available around the clock, but physicians may only be called in when a patient arrives.

2. Basic Emergency Department: This is the most common type of ED, meeting minimum standards that include 24-hour nursing services, physician availability, diagnostic capabilities, and on-call subspecialty services.

3. Comprehensive Emergency Department: Relatively rare, these EDs are usually affiliated with teaching hospitals. They provide extensive services with specialized physicians available on-site for high-volume patient care. These EDs support complex cases and often function in

academic medical centers (Office of Statewide Health Planning and Development [OSHPD], 2012).

The level of services provided is determined by state regulations, and requirements may differ from state to state.

Trauma Designation: Levels I-IV

Trauma care facilities are categorized into levels based on the resources and services they provide. These designations, ranging from Level I to Level IV (and sometimes Level V), are determined by states and must comply with specified criteria.

Trauma Systems and Collaboration: A trauma system is a network of facilities that works together to provide coordinated care for trauma patients. This system is designed based on geographic regions, population density, and facility resources, rather than political boundaries. The goal is to ensure patients receive care in the most appropriate facility based on the severity of their injuries.

Levels of Trauma Centers:

Level IV: These centers provide the most basic trauma services, typically with a general ED and trauma surgeon on call.

Level III: Level III centers offer more comprehensive trauma services, including continuous coverage for orthopedic surgeries but may lack specialized pelvic fracture surgical services.

Level II: These centers offer a broad range of surgical services, including neuro and maxillofacial surgery, and can handle all but the most complex trauma cases.

Level I: The highest level of trauma care, with specialized services often available on-site. These facilities also provide services like burn units, organ transplants, and complex limb surgeries. Level I centers are frequently affiliated with academic medical institutions.

Trauma centers are designated by states, but organizations like the American College of Surgeons (ACS) verify that facilities meet the necessary standards for their trauma level. Verification by independent bodies ensures the accuracy of the designation and adherence to evidence-based practices. Verification standards are updated regularly by organizations like the ACS.

Trauma Center Verification and State Designation: States delegate regulatory authority for trauma centers to agencies like the Local Emergency Medical Services Agency (LEMSA). These agencies oversee compliance with state and regional trauma system requirements. While states grant designations, verification by third-party organizations like the ACS ensures that facilities meet resource standards, offering a higher level of confidence in the facility's capabilities.

Pediatric Emergency Medical Services Readiness

The need for pediatric emergency care has been recognized in various reports, such as the Institute of Medicine's 1993 publication, which noted that many EDs lacked the training and equipment necessary to meet pediatric care standards. The response has been to implement certification programs like the Emergency Department Approved for Pediatrics (EDAP) and Pediatric Trauma Center verification. Professional organizations, such as the American Heart Association and the Emergency Nurses Association, offer training programs like Pediatric Advanced Life Support (PALS) to standardize pediatric care practices.

Pediatric patients make up approximately 25%-35% of ED visits (Schappert & Bhuiya, 2012). EDs aiming to specialize in pediatric care should invest in training, equipment, and certifications such as PALS or Emergency

Nursing Pediatric Course (ENPC) to provide optimal care.

## Geriatric Emergency Departments: Specialization and Standards

As the geriatric population continues to grow, there is an increasing need for specialized care within emergency departments. Consensus guidelines from multiple medical organizations emphasize the importance of adapting EDs to meet the unique needs of elderly patients. This includes specific staffing protocols, physical environment modifications, and training for healthcare providers.

Key Recommendations for Geriatric EDs:

Staffing Protocols: Geriatric-trained providers, including physicians, nurses, and support staff, should be on hand. A designated geriatric emergency medicine director and nurse manager are essential.

Discharge Protocols: These should include adaptations for elderly patients, such as large-print discharge instructions and clear communication with family members and caregivers to reduce hospital readmission rates.

Equipment and Supplies: Facilities should be equipped with geriatric-friendly furniture, such as easily accessible gurneys, fall mats, and appropriate lighting.

Quality Improvement Plans: EDs should track metrics like geriatric patient volume, admission rates, and readmission rates, implementing interventions when necessary to maintain high standards of care.

Career Opportunities: The proportion of geriatric patients varies depending on local demographics. EDs specializing in geriatric care may attract a higher percentage of elderly patients, providing ample opportunities for career growth in this field. Institutions emphasizing geriatric care are more likely to benefit from a competitive edge in attracting patients, particularly in regions with an aging population (American College of Emergency Physicians, American Geriatrics Society, Emergency Nurses Association, Society for Academic Emergency Medicine, 2013).

Disease-Specific Centers, Certifications, and Designations

The positive outcomes associated with trauma-center designations have led to a growing demand for other disease-specific designations, certifications, and verifications. Emergency Medical Systems (EMS) are well-suited to direct patients to facilities that are most equipped to provide optimal care for specific conditions.

Disease-specific certifications are expanding within both Emergency Departments (EDs) and across entire hospitals. EMS regulations often include protocols that bypass the closest facility to ensure patients are transported to the hospital best prepared to manage their specific condition. Examples of these designations include Chest Pain Centers and Stroke Centers, but many others are emerging. The resources available under these certifications can vary depending on the organization supporting the designation.

These certifications and designations can reveal a hospital's focus and resource allocation. For example, The Joint Commission offers both basic and advanced certifications for a variety of disease processes, such as chest pain, orthopedic and spinal surgeries, and sepsis, among others. Additionally, the American Heart Association and the Society of Chest Pain Centers offer certifications for cardiac and stroke care. These certifications allow facilities to benchmark their practices against others, improve their care delivery, and advertise their specialized services. Consumers can trust that these facilities are engaged in providing highly organized care, validated by external oversight and ensuring that the care exceeds the minimum requirements mandated by state laws.

## Chest Pain Center and Other Disease-Specific Certifications

Certifications, such as those for Chest Pain Centers, ensure that the facility is equipped to deliver the best possible care for that specific condition. These designations assure consumers and healthcare professionals that the facility meets industry standards for diagnostic capabilities, staffing levels, and protocols. Certified centers operate under established processes that allow for timely recognition and treatment of conditions such as acute coronary syndromes. In order to advertise a trademarked designation like "Chest Pain Center," a facility must pay for, and submit to, regular surveys by an external agency. These agencies typically require recurrent disease-specific education for the staff, ensuring that knowledge is kept up to date. Organizations that pursue such certifications demonstrate a commitment to quality beyond basic licensing requirements, creating an environment that fosters professional growth.

For a hospital to be designated as a Chest Pain Center by the Society of Cardiovascular Patient Care, the following requirements are typically mandated (UNC Healthcare, 2012):

The hospital must implement a community education program focused on recognizing heart attack symptoms and the importance of immediate medical care.

The hospital must integrate Emergency Department (ED) services with pre-hospital services to ensure timely transport and care for patients with chest pain.

Written protocols must exist to allow for the prompt recognition of acute coronary syndromes.

The hospital must have comprehensive diagnostic capabilities, such as biomarkers, 12-lead ECG interpretation, and stress testing for assessing patients with chest pain.

The hospital must implement a continuous process improvement plan for evaluating and enhancing the care provided to chest pain patients.

Staff involved in patient care must be properly credentialed and regularly trained.

The hospital's administration must demonstrate a commitment to maintaining Chest Pain Center accreditation.

Clear and accessible signage must be provided to help patients and pre-hospital providers locate the center.

Career Context for Certified Facilities

Facilities with disease-specific certifications focus on achieving measurable outcomes and improving operations. This is often accomplished through education and regular performance reviews. For example, a facility with a cardiac-designated ED and an interventional catheterization lab provides valuable opportunities for nurses passionate about treating patients with acute myocardial infarctions.

Free-Standing Emergency Departments

Free-standing Emergency Departments (EDs) offer competitive advantages in states where they are licensed. These facilities provide critical care for time-sensitive conditions and can improve care delivery by reducing door-to-doctor times, particularly in areas experiencing high patient volumes. Unlike urgent care centers, free-standing EDs offer comprehensive services, including radiology and laboratory testing. However, they are not directly connected to hospitals, so patients who require inpatient services are transferred to a nearby hospital. While this model is not universally licensed across all states, it can offer high-quality, timely care and improve patient outcomes, particularly in critical conditions such as embolic stroke.

Career Context for Free-Standing EDs

Free-standing EDs provide an exciting opportunity for healthcare professionals who enjoy rapid intervention and transferring high-acuity patients to more specialized hospitals.

Urgent Care Centers

Urgent care centers, which are often stand-alone facilities, cater to non-life-threatening conditions such as minor fractures and illnesses. Unlike hospitals, they are not subject to rigorous licensing requirements, though they may be overseen by hospital regulations if they are affiliated. These centers bridge the gap between primary care and emergency care, providing services without the need for appointments and offering basic diagnostic capabilities. However, any need for inpatient care or specialized consultation requires transfer to a hospital. Working in an urgent care center allows exposure to outpatient medical practice and patient care.

Career Context for Urgent Care Centers

Urgent care centers offer a lower-intensity environment compared to EDs, with shorter patient stays and fewer nursing interventions. Healthcare professionals in these settings will gain experience in episodic care, typically dealing with lower acuity cases.

Lantern Award

The Lantern Award, bestowed by the Emergency Nurses Association (ENA), is given to EDs that demonstrate exceptional performance across leadership, clinical practice, education, advocacy, and research. Only about 1% of EDs in the U.S. receive this prestigious recognition. To qualify, a facility must undergo a survey to ensure it meets the standards outlined by the ENA. Reapplication is required annually to maintain the designation, making it a mark of sustained excellence.

Career Context for Lantern Award Designated EDs

Working in an ED with a Lantern Award designation means being part of a team that strives for excellence in emergency care. These facilities demonstrate a commitment to providing outstanding emergency services, offering an ideal environment for professionals who value innovation and high standards.

Magnet Designation

Magnet® status is granted to hospitals that demonstrate exceptional nursing care across a broad range of focus areas. Awarded by the American Nurses Credentialing Center (ANCC), it recognizes facilities where nursing staff are empowered and committed to evidence-based practice. Magnet hospitals excel in quality care, professional satisfaction, and shared governance, offering an environment conducive to nursing leadership and professional growth.

Career Context for Magnet Facilities

Magnet hospitals offer high rates of nursing satisfaction and are known for attracting top nursing talent due to their commitment to quality care and nursing-centered environments. For nurses, working in a Magnet facility is often seen as an opportunity to thrive in a collaborative and professionally fulfilling setting.

Summary

The diversity of emergency nursing environments reflects the wide range of patient needs. From critical access EDs to university teaching hospital trauma centers, every facility offers a unique opportunity for professional growth. As nurses progress in their careers, transitioning to different environments provides new challenges and learning opportunities. Each department, while serving similar patient populations, uses a different set of resources, allowing professional nurses to continually advance their skills and knowledge.

References

1. American College of Emergency Physicians, American Geriatrics Society, Emergency Nurses Association, & Society for Academic Emergency Medicine. (2013). Geriatric emergency department guidelines. Retrieved from

http://www.acep.org/workarea/DownloadAsset.aspx?id=95365

2. American College of Surgeons. (2014). Resources for optimal care of the injured patient (6th ed.; M. F. Rotondo, C. Cribari, & S. R. Smith, Eds.). Chicago, IL: American College of Surgeons.

3. American Nurses Credentialing Center (ANCC). (2015). System eligibility requirements. Retrieved from http://www.nursecredentialing.org/SysEligibilityRequirements

4. American Trauma Society (ATS). (n.d.). Trauma center levels explained. Retrieved from http://www.amtrauma.org/?page=traumalevels

5. Catholic Health Association of the United States. (2015, January). Facts and statistics: Catholic health care in the

United States. Retrieved from https://www.chausa.org/about/about/facts-statistics

6. Centers for Disease Control and Prevention (CDC). (2015, April 29). Emergency department visits. Retrieved from http://www.cdc.gov/nchs/fastats/emergency-department.htm

7. Centers for Medicare and Medicaid Services (CMS). (2013, April 10). Outlier payments. Retrieved from https://www.cms.gov/Medicare/Medicare-Fee-for-Service-Payment/AcuteInpatientPPS/outlier.html

8. Department of Health and Human Services, Centers for Medicare and Medicaid Services. (2014, September). Critical Access Hospital. Retrieved from http://www.cms.gov/Outreach-and-Education/Medicare-Learning-Network-MLN/M

LNProducts/downloads/CritAccessHospfctsht.pdf

9. Emergency Nurses Association (ENA). (2015). Lantern Award. Retrieved from https://www.ena.org/practice-research/Practice/LanternAward/Pages/default.aspx

10. Internal Revenue Service (IRS). (2015). New requirements for 501(c)(3) hospitals under the Affordable Care Act. Retrieved from http://www.irs.gov/Charities-&-Non-Profits/Charitable-Organizations/New-Requirements-for-501(c)(3)-Hospitals-Under-the-Affordable-Care-Act

11. International Committee of the Red Cross (ICRC). (2015). Practice relating to Rule 35. Hospital and safety zones and neutralized zones. Retrieved from https://www.icrc.org/customary-ihl/eng/docs/v2_rul_rule35

12. Millman, M. (1993). Access to healthcare in America. Washington, DC: National Academies Press.

13. Office of Statewide Health Planning and Development (OSHPD). (2010). Emergency room hospitals. Retrieved from http://gis.oshpd.ca.gov/atlas/topics/er_dashboard

14. Pediatric Readiness Project. (n.d.). Average pediatric readiness scores. Retrieved from http://www.pediatricreadiness.org/State_Results/Average_Scores.aspx

15. Schappert, S. M., & Bhuiya, F. (2012, March 1). Availability of pediatric services and equipment in emergency departments: United States, 2006. Retrieved from http://www.cdc.gov/nchs/data/nhsr/nhsr047.pdf

16. UNC Healthcare. (2012, November 8). Working towards chest pain center accreditation. Retrieved from http://news.unchealthcare.org/som-vital-signs/2012/nov8/working-towards-chest-pain-center-accreditation

## Chapter 4
## The Role of the Emergency Nurse in Triage

Introduction to Triage in Emergency Nursing

Triage is a critical component of emergency nursing, a responsibility that distinguishes emergency nurses from their counterparts in other clinical settings. While nurses across various healthcare environments perform assessments and prioritize patient care, the triage nurse faces unique challenges in managing complex patient evaluations. These decisions, made independently, can have significant consequences for the patient's outcome and for the overall operation of the emergency department (ED). This chapter outlines the essential role of the triage nurse and the fundamental principles guiding the triage process.

The triage nurse's duties require an understanding of both the functional responsibilities and the underlying principles of triage. The nature of triage in emergency settings necessitates a structured and standardized approach to ensure the delivery of high-quality care. According to the Emergency Nurses Association (ENA) Standards of Practice, the emergency nurse is tasked with evaluating patients and determining the priority of care based on physical, psychological, and social needs, in addition to factors that influence the flow through the emergency care system (ENA, 2011a).

Defining Triage

The term "triage" comes from the French verb trier, meaning "to sort" or "to choose." It was first used in a medical context in the 1930s within the military. As healthcare shifted from house calls to hospital-based care, emergency departments saw an influx of patients, necessitating a system to prioritize those in greatest need. By the mid-20th century, this system began to be adopted from military models to civilian hospitals, ensuring timely care for the most critically ill. Today, triage remains a core practice in virtually every U.S. ED, though it is a skill mainly exclusive to emergency nursing. Poorly executed triage can have dire consequences for patient care.

Triage is defined as the process of assigning urgency to illnesses or injuries in order to prioritize treatment. This dynamic process ensures that patients receive care from the appropriate healthcare provider at the right time, utilizing limited resources effectively.

The Legal Context of Triage
The Emergency Medical Treatment and Labor Act (EMTALA), passed in the 1980s, addressed concerns over "patient dumping," ensuring that emergency departments provide care regardless of a patient's ability to pay. EMTALA mandates a medical screening examination (MSE) to determine the existence of an emergency medical condition. This law significantly

influenced triage practices by making clear the distinction between the triage process and the MSE (see Chapter 12 for more on risk management and quality issues).

Qualifications of the Triage Nurse

Triage nurses must be prepared for the high-stakes decision-making that impacts both patient outcomes and departmental efficiency. These nurses often work in isolated areas, making decisions independently while coordinating the overall functioning of the ED. Given these demands, it is crucial that only qualified individuals are assigned triage duties.

Although some nurses may rotate through triage as part of their general ED responsibilities, the triage role requires specific qualifications. These include:

Registered nurse status, completion of a standardized triage education program with both theoretical and clinical components

Certification in CPR and Advanced Life Support (ALS)

Completion of specialized courses like the Emergency Nursing Pediatric Course (ENPC) and Trauma Nursing Core Course (TNCC)

Certification as a Certified Emergency Nurse (CEN) or Certified Pediatric Emergency Nurse (CPEN) is preferred.

Personal attributes critical for triage nurses include strong communication and critical thinking skills, the ability to perform rapid assessments, and the ability to make accurate decisions in high-pressure situations. Triage nurses must also work well within interdisciplinary teams and maintain a patient-centered, empathetic approach (ENA, 2011b).

Critical Thinking in Triage

Effective triage relies heavily on the nurse's ability to engage in critical thinking. Important qualities include:

Inquisitive: Asking focused questions to gather relevant information from patients and caregivers.

Systematic: Ensuring a thorough collection of patient data to avoid missing critical details.

Analytical: Anticipating potential changes in a patient's condition based on current symptoms.

Truth-seeking: Approaching each situation with objectivity, especially when sensitive issues like non-accidental trauma are suspected.

Open-mindedness: Avoiding bias and stereotyping, which may influence clinical decisions.

Self-confidence: Being decisive in high-pressure situations while trusting one's clinical judgment.

Maturity: Remaining open to revising clinical decisions as new information becomes available.

## Triage Systems

Triage systems provide a structured framework for prioritizing patient care. While triage acuity scales assist in sorting patients by urgency, the triage system itself encompasses broader operational goals, ensuring that patients are seen in an efficient and organized manner. Historically, several types of triage systems have been developed, each with varying degrees of complexity and resource utilization.

### 1. Traffic Director System

This basic triage method involves minimal patient assessment, typically only identifying the chief complaint. Non-medical staff often carry out this system, which lacks the detail and rigor required for proper triage. This approach is discouraged due to legal concerns, including the violation of EMTALA requirements.

2. Spot Check Triage

In spot check triage, a registered nurse gathers the patient's history and performs basic assessments. The priority is given to the most critically ill patients. While this system uses established protocols, inconsistencies in staff experience can lead to variable decision-making. Documentation and reassessment processes are often minimal in this approach, which can lead to inefficiencies.

3. Comprehensive Triage

Comprehensive triage is the most advanced and preferred method, involving a thorough assessment of subjective and objective data, including medical history, psychosocial factors, and overall health status. This method ensures that patients are classified accurately and receive timely care. Comprehensive triage utilizes written protocols, diagnostic tests, and established guidelines to manage patient flow and decision-making effectively.

Implementing a Triage System
To optimize the effectiveness of any triage system, several key components must be in place:

Physical environment: A well-organized triage area with the necessary tools and space for assessments.

Documentation: Effective documentation tools are essential to ensure that all triage decisions are accurately recorded and that patient care is coordinated properly.

A rapid triage assessment should be completed within 60-90 seconds, with more detailed assessments taking 2-5 minutes. Ensuring that these timelines are met is crucial for efficient ED operations. Lack of support systems, including proper tools and protocols, can hinder the triage process and compromise patient care.

The Triage Process: A Systematic Approach to Emergency Care

The triage process is an essential aspect of emergency care, determining how patients are prioritized based on the severity of their condition. While the triage system outlines the overall framework, the triage process is the way in which nurses and healthcare professionals carry out the steps within this system. A well-organized triage process ensures that patient data is collected systematically and documented accurately.

As McNair (2006) states, "Triage is not a PLACE... it is a PROCESS" (p. 11). Triage serves as one of the critical "point-of-entry" processes within the emergency department (ED). Whether patients arrive by walking, ambulance, or private vehicle, they must be assessed, prioritized, and assigned appropriate care based on their acuity and disposition. This process uses the nursing model to evaluate and care for patients. The triage assessment can be either rapid or comprehensive, but in all cases, it follows a structured decision-making process that includes an across-the-room assessment, patient interview, physical examination, and final triage decision regarding the patient's acuity and necessary disposition (McNair, 2012).

Steps of the Triage Assessment Process

1. Critical Look (Across the Room Assessment): Before engaging with the patient, the triage nurse makes initial observations from a distance to assess the patient's condition. This involves looking at factors such as posture, facial expression, and method of arrival.

2. Chief Complaint: The nurse asks the patient about their primary reason for seeking care, which can guide the next steps of the assessment. This is vital in cases requiring immediate attention, as the nature of the complaint may dictate urgency.

3. Rapid Triage Assessment: If the patient meets the criteria for immediate care (such as obvious signs of severe illness), a rapid assessment is performed to decide the appropriate placement. This includes noting vital signs and initial physical findings.

4. Comprehensive Triage Assessment: If the patient does not meet immediate care criteria, a more thorough assessment is conducted. This helps to evaluate the patient's condition more fully and assign the appropriate level of care.

5. Acuity Level and Disposition: Based on the assessment, the nurse determines the patient's acuity level, which informs the urgency and type of care required. This is documented using a specific triage acuity scale.

6. Nursing Interventions and Diagnostics: The nurse initiates necessary interventions, which may include administering medications, conducting diagnostic tests, or preparing the

patient for further treatment based on established protocols or under the direction of a licensed independent practitioner (LIP).

7. Reassessment: Regular reassessment is crucial to ensure the patient's condition is accurately monitored and appropriate care is provided throughout the process. This involves reviewing changes in the patient's status and updating the triage decision as needed.

The Critical Look (Across the Room Assessment)

The "critical look" or initial observation allows the triage nurse to gain valuable insights even before interacting directly with the patient. The nurse uses all available senses during this assessment:

Sight: Visual cues such as skin color, facial expressions, and posture can suggest the severity of the condition. Observing how the patient arrives and interacts with others can also provide important context.

Hearing: Sounds such as labored breathing, coughing, or altered speech may indicate more severe conditions and help prioritize care.

Smell: Unusual odors, such as fruity breath (indicating potential ketoacidosis) or the smell of alcohol or coal gas, can offer diagnostic clues.

Touch: Physical contact allows the nurse to gauge skin temperature, moisture, and other tactile clues that inform the patient's status.

Intuition: Triage nurses should trust their instincts, as an "unsettling" feeling may indicate a need for heightened urgency.

Eliciting the Chief Complaint

Once the initial assessment is made, the next step is to obtain the patient's chief complaint. This is a critical piece of information, as it often directly influences the urgency of the situation. In some cases, the nature of the complaint itself—such as chest pain or severe trauma—may necessitate immediate intervention, bypassing further assessment.

Rapid and Comprehensive Triage Assessment

A comprehensive triage assessment requires both objective and subjective information. Triage nurses must ask the right questions in the right way to ensure accuracy. Open-ended questions are particularly valuable in reducing errors and improving diagnostic accuracy during patient interviews. This communication skill must be learned and refined but can significantly improve triage decisions.

In addition to assessing the current issue, the nurse may also gather relevant background information, such as the patient's medical history, allergies, and medication usage. This information is essential for making informed triage decisions. A simple mnemonic (Gurney & Westergard, 2014) can help remember key history components:

S: Symptoms associated with the current injury or illness

A: Allergies and tetanus status

M: Medication history

P: Past medical history

L: Last oral intake or menstrual period

E: Events leading to the illness or injury

While a detailed history is useful, it should be limited to what is pertinent to the immediate triage decision, as time is often of the essence.

Physical Examination and Documentation

A brief physical examination is often necessary as part of the triage process. The nurse should examine the area of concern, making comparisons where applicable. Symmetry, tenderness, and other findings can offer valuable clues about the severity of the condition.

Effective documentation is also a cornerstone of triage. Clear and concise recording of findings ensures that relevant data is captured and can be quickly referenced by other healthcare providers. Good documentation is characterized by brevity and clarity, which enables the swift delivery of care and reduces the risk of errors.

Triage Acuity Assessment and Documentation

Triage, the process of categorizing patients based on the urgency of their medical needs, plays a crucial role in managing emergency department (ED) care. An essential part of this process is determining the acuity level of each patient, which helps prioritize treatment. However, there is currently no standardized national triage scale in the United States, leading to variations in the systems used across different healthcare institutions. These systems, though not universally uniform, must allow for flexibility and integrate both objective and subjective assessments. Consequently, assigning an acuity level should not be viewed as an exact science, but rather a dynamic decision-making process, where triage nurses apply their clinical judgment.

Key Clinical Prioritization Strategies

To ensure appropriate care, triage nurses utilize several clinical prioritization strategies:

Systemic over local: Treating the whole body before focusing on localized issues.

Life before limb: Prioritizing life-threatening conditions over less severe limb injuries.

Acute over chronic pain: Addressing urgent, acute conditions before chronic ones.

These principles guide nurses in making rapid decisions, balancing urgent care with necessary resource allocation.

## National Triage System: A Work in Progress

Since 2005, the Emergency Nurses Association (ENA) and the American College of Emergency Physicians (ACEP) have advocated for a national five-level triage system. Although no specific system has been endorsed, they support the adoption of a statistically reliable and valid system for consistency across institutions. In the absence of a national standard, hospitals are free to select the acuity system that best suits their needs. However, it is crucial that staff are adequately trained to apply the chosen system consistently.

Examples of Triage Systems

1. Canadian Triage and Acuity Scale (CTAS): The CTAS is a well-developed triage system that emphasizes the symptomatic presentation of patients rather than their likely diagnosis. It assigns acuity based on key symptoms, categorizing patients from resuscitation (Level I) to non-urgent (Level V). For example, a patient with chest pain and associated symptoms may be assigned a higher acuity level, while chest pain without these indicators would be categorized as lower acuity. The CTAS provides operational benchmarks, such as recommended time frames for patient care (e.g., emergent care within 15 minutes), and tools like fractile responses to measure performance against these standards.

2. Emergency Severity Index (ESI): The ESI is a five-level triage system that evaluates both the patient's acuity and their expected resource

needs. Developed by Drs. Richard Wuerz and David Eitel, this system helps streamline patient care by assessing the urgency of medical conditions and the resources required for treatment. It is widely used in U.S. emergency departments, with updates and guidance available in the ESI Implementation Handbook.

3. Australasian Triage Scale (ATS) and Manchester Triage System (MTS): Both the ATS and MTS are internationally recognized five-level systems that use symptom-driven algorithms for nurse-led triage. The ATS focuses on a series of questioning steps to determine acuity, while the MTS employs flow charts based on over 50 clinical symptoms to guide decision-making.

Initiating Nursing Interventions and Diagnostics

Beyond assigning triage acuity, nurses also play an active role in patient care, often initiating interventions that are essential to stabilizing the patient. These interventions can begin as soon as the patient arrives, even before a definitive diagnosis is made.

1. Rapid Medical Evaluation (RME): In some settings, patients are kept near the entry point in a Rapid Medical Evaluation area, where a licensed practitioner performs preliminary assessments and orders diagnostics. This approach reduces delays and facilitates quicker decision-making regarding further treatment or admission.

2. Advanced Triage Protocols (ATP): Nurses are sometimes required to implement advanced triage protocols that involve standing orders or clinical pathways. These protocols allow nurses to initiate specific treatments or diagnostic tests based on established guidelines. However, the use of ATPs requires nurses to be highly skilled and up-to-date with current practices. Ensuring that all nurses are trained in these protocols is vital for maintaining consistency and patient safety.

3. First Aid and Comfort Measures: Basic interventions like pain management, splinting, and applying ice should not be overlooked. These foundational measures are essential in providing immediate relief and stabilizing patients. In fact, timely first aid can reduce the need for more advanced interventions and improve overall patient satisfaction. For instance, a patient with a shoulder dislocation may experience significant pain relief from proper splinting and ice application, potentially reducing their acuity level.

4. Assessing and Adjusting Acuity: Nurses are often the first to identify changes in a patient's condition, which may require adjustments to their acuity level. A study by McQueen and Gay (2010) found that many patients with acute traumatic shoulder dislocation did not receive appropriate pain management, leading to delays in diagnosis and treatment. This highlights the critical role of the triage nurse in setting the trajectory for the patient's care.

Challenges and Compliance Issues in Triage

Despite the availability of triage protocols, studies have shown significant variability in their implementation. For example, research by Fosnocht (2007) found that compliance with triage pain protocols varied widely among nurses, ranging from 8% to 96%. This inconsistency suggests that more robust training and ongoing education are necessary to ensure protocols are followed correctly. Nurses must be not only experienced but also clinically current to apply triage protocols effectively.

Moreover, some nurses may be encouraged to act before obtaining a physician's order, which can lead to potential legal and professional issues. It is essential that all interventions align with established protocols and that any deviations are clearly justified.

Patient Disposition in Emergency Departments: An Evidence-Based Approach

Triage decisions in the emergency department (ED) are critical not only for determining the urgency of patient care but also for managing the flow, order, and safety of the entire ED environment. Traditional triage often has been misunderstood as a rigid, sequential process, where patients are lined up and seen in the order they arrive or after completing several mandatory steps, such as providing a chief complaint and undergoing full registration and assessment. This approach fails to consider the dynamic nature of triage, which must be flexible and adaptive to meet the varying clinical needs and operational constraints of the ED.

In recent years, significant advancements in triage protocols have emphasized the need for a more responsive system. Triage should no longer be viewed as a static process. Modern triage requires clinical judgment, with healthcare professionals making real-time decisions based on patient acuity, resources, and the operational status of the ED. Effective triage incorporates a variety of strategies, such as "pull-until-full" or "split-flow," designed to manage patient flow efficiently. These strategies aim to streamline patient movement from the waiting area to treatment beds, although, if not executed properly, they can create new bottlenecks in patient care, such as overcrowded treatment areas or insufficient nursing resources. Therefore, it is crucial that EDs establish specific criteria for when to prioritize immediate bedding or direct patients to treatment areas, particularly during periods of high volume.

Ambulance Triage and Pre-Treatment Assessment

Patients arriving by ambulance should also undergo a triage assessment before being assigned to a treatment bed. This assessment may be conducted in areas separate from traditional triage zones, often by a charge nurse or bed flow coordinator trained in triage protocols. In cases of severe illness or injury, the assessment can rely on the EMS report to determine triage priority quickly. However, if the assessment reveals lower acuity, the patient may be placed in the queue with other ambulatory patients, as mode of transportation should not dictate bed assignment.

It is important to remember that critically ill or injured patients, whether arriving by ambulance or private vehicle, should be triaged appropriately according to the severity of their condition. Triage is a process, not a location, and every patient—whether they are trauma patients or those with other critical conditions—must be evaluated and integrated into the ED intake process.

Common Pitfalls in Triage and Strategies for Prevention

Triage nurses must be aware of several potential pitfalls that can impair decision-making and negatively impact patient outcomes:

1. Focusing Only on the Presenting Complaint: While the presenting complaint is important, it is crucial not to overlook the broader clinical picture. Assumptions based solely on initial symptoms can lead to missed diagnoses. Nurses should always consider the possibility of underlying issues and gather a comprehensive history.

2. Failure to Elicit the Right Information: Triage nurses are the first line of assessment and must often rely on patient history, which may not always be clear or complete. It is essential to ask open-ended questions and pursue further details when symptoms or complaints are ambiguous. If the clinical picture remains unclear, it may be prudent to assign a higher triage priority until further assessment can be made.

3. Loss of Objectivity: Frequent patients or those with a history of chronic conditions may not

always present with urgent needs, but it is essential to maintain an unbiased approach. Returning patients, especially those visiting within 72 hours of a previous visit, require careful attention to ensure that their current concerns are properly evaluated and not dismissed based on prior visits.

4. Distraction Due to Multiple Patients: During busy periods, the influx of patients can be overwhelming, but it is important to focus on the most urgent cases first. Triage staff should apply a systematic approach to ensure that patient needs are prioritized based on acuity. The following steps can help maintain focus and efficiency:

Assess ABCs (Airway, Breathing, Circulation): Regularly scan the room to ensure that all patients have an intact airway, are breathing, and do not exhibit signs of distress (e.g., pallor, diaphoresis). These patients should be prioritized.

Elicit Chief Complaints: Quickly identify the chief complaint of each patient, distinguishing between patients and their accompanying family members. This helps in categorizing patients and deciding who requires immediate attention.

Determine Priority for Comprehensive Assessment: Based on the initial findings, decide who requires immediate intervention and who can wait for a more thorough triage assessment.

## Challenges in Emergency Department Triage: Stress, Communication, and Equipment Usage

### Stress and Isolation in Triage Roles

Triage in the emergency department (ED) is often one of the most isolated areas, with limited resources and support. Nurses working in this area are frequently faced with a high patient-to-nurse ratio, minimal assistance, and few breaks. This isolation, compounded by a lack of relief, can result in significant stress, which in turn affects critical thinking and decision-making. Quality care requires that nurses take breaks to recharge and address basic biological needs, such as bathroom breaks or snacks. It is essential that triage be staffed by trained personnel rather than volunteers or administrative staff to ensure continuous patient care and staff well-being. Protecting the triage nurse ultimately ensures that the entire ED is well-served. For more on self-care, refer to Chapter 6.

Improper Use of Medical Equipment
Correct usage of medical equipment is crucial for accurate diagnosis and patient outcomes. For instance, the correct size of blood pressure cuffs must be used, as improper sizing can lead to incorrect readings. Similarly, tympanic thermometers, while commonly used, may not be appropriate for all patients, such as small children, the elderly, or those exposed to extreme temperatures. Pulse oximetry is another tool that requires careful interpretation. Conditions like hypothermia or alkalosis can skew results,

leading to falsely high oxygen saturation levels. This phenomenon occurs because the oxyhemoglobin dissociation curve shifts, preventing effective oxygen delivery to tissues despite a normal oxygen saturation reading. Moreover, abnormal hemoglobins (such as carboxyhemoglobin or methemoglobinemia) can interfere with pulse oximetry accuracy, potentially leading to misleading clinical decisions.

Communication in the Emergency Department
Effective communication is essential in improving patient satisfaction in the ED, particularly regarding wait times. Research indicates that it is not the length of the wait that causes dissatisfaction, but rather the psychological aspects of the experience. Providing clear, timely information and addressing patient concerns about wait times can significantly improve their perception of care. A study by Thompson et al. (1996) demonstrated that managing expectations, offering information, and delivering care with empathy

are more effective strategies for patient satisfaction than simply reducing wait times.

Conclusion

Triage represents a critical and highly autonomous role in the emergency department, where nurses apply their clinical expertise, critical thinking, and compassion to make life-saving decisions. It is essential for nurses to take care of themselves and use equipment correctly to ensure that patients receive the best care possible. Furthermore, strong communication skills are vital to managing patient expectations and improving satisfaction in the ED.

References

1. Canadian Association of Emergency Physicians (CAEP). (2008). Revisions to the Canadian Emergency Department triage and acuity. CTAS guide to implementation.

Retrieved from http://caep.ca/resources/ctas/implementation-guidelines

2. Canadian Association of Emergency Physicians (CAEP). (2013). CTAS implementation guidelines, 2013 revisions to CTAS guidelines. Retrieved from http://caep.ca/resources/ctas#guidelines

3. Emergency Nurses Association (ENA). (2011a). Emergency nursing: Scope and standards of practice. Des Plaines, IL: Emergency Nurses Association.

4. Emergency Nurses Association (ENA). (2011b). Triage qualifications position statement. Des Plaines, IL: Emergency Nurses Association.

5. Emergency Nurses Association (ENA). (2015, January). Course in Advanced Trauma Nursing II: A conceptual approach to injury and illness. Des Plaines, IL: Emergency Nurses Association.

6. Facione, P. A. (2011). Critical thinking: What it is and why it counts (2011 update). Retrieved May 14, 2011, from http://www.insightassessment.com/pdf_files/What&Why2010.pdf

7. Fernandes, C. G. (2005). Five-level triage: A report from the ACEP/ENA five-level triage task force. Journal of Emergency Nursing, 31(1), 39–50.

8. Fosnocht, D. E. (2007). Use of a triage pain protocol in the ED. The American Journal of Emergency Medicine, 25(7), 791–793.

9. Gilboy, N. T. (2012). Emergency Severity Index (ESI): A triage tool for emergency department care, Version 4. Rockville, MD: U.S. Department of Health and Human Services, Agency for Healthcare Research and Quality (AHRQ).

10. Gurney, D., & Westergard, A. M. (2014). Initial assessment. In E. N. Association, Trauma nursing core course (7th ed., pp. 39–54). Des Plaines, IL: Emergency Nurses Association.

11. Heisenberg, W. (1962). Physics and philosophy: The revolution in modern science. New York, NY: Harper & Row Publishers.

12. McCallum, L., & Higgins, D. (2012). Measuring body temperature. Nursing Times, 108(45), 20–22.

13. McNair, R. (2006). Patient safety through managing triage and emergency department workflow. Triage First Education; Comprehensive emergency department triage course workbook. Fairview, NC: Triage First, Inc.

14. McNair, R. (2012). ED triage systematics: ED triage comprehensive course. Fairview, NC: Triage First, Inc.

15. McQueen, C. G., & Gay, K. J. (2010). Retrospective audit to triage of acute traumatic shoulder dislocation by emergency nurses. Journal of Emergency Nursing, 36(1), 21–25.

16. Thompson, D., Yarnold, P., Williams, D., & Adams, S. (1996). Effects of actual waiting time, information delivery, and expressive quality on patient satisfaction in the emergency department. Annals of Emergency Medicine, 28, 657–665.

## Chapter 5
## Risk Management and Quality Issues in Emergency Nursing

The emergency department (ED) is uniquely positioned within the hospital, characterized by unpredictable challenges, high patient volume, and the need for continuous availability. Unlike other departments, the ED operates 24/7 and handles patients of all ages, conditions, and levels of acuity without controlling their number or timing of arrival. This requires emergency nurses to exhibit adaptability and vigilance in identifying and addressing risks to patient safety proactively. Mastering the principles of professional liability and employing tools to mitigate risks is essential for enhancing patient care and minimizing legal exposure.

A comprehensive understanding of hospital protocols, legal and regulatory frameworks, and evidence-based best practices is critical. This chapter outlines the interplay between professional liability, quality improvement, and patient safety in emergency nursing.

Acceptable Standards of Care

The Institute of Medicine (IOM) report, To Err Is Human: Building a Safer Health System (2000), estimated that preventable medical errors contribute to 44,000–98,000 annual hospital deaths. The report emphasized reducing preventable errors by 50% within five years and highlighted a national focus on improving healthcare safety (Kohn, Corrigan, & Donaldson, 2000).

The Joint Commission took this further in 1998 by issuing its first Sentinel Event Alert, urging healthcare facilities to conduct root cause analyses for serious incidents leading to patient harm. These analyses identified trends in sentinel events, which are shared publicly to encourage adoption of preventive measures. The Joint Commission also introduced National

Patient Safety Goals in 2002, many of which have since become standard care practices.

Multiple organizations contribute to ongoing patient safety research and policy development, including:

Lucian Leape Institute of the National Patient Safety Foundation (2007)

Agency for Healthcare Research and Quality (AHRQ, 1989)

Emergency Care Research Institute (ECRI, 1968)

Risk Management in the Emergency Department

Risk management in clinical settings involves safeguarding organizational assets by enhancing patient and workplace safety. It includes addressing legal, regulatory, and operational risks. For instance, between 1991 and 2013, ED visits rose by 45 million, while 668 EDs closed due to unsustainable operational costs (American Hospital Association [AHA], 2015). This disproportion has strained the remaining EDs, which continue to serve as safety nets for patients lacking alternative care options.

The Affordable Care Act (ACA) has attempted to redirect patients to primary care providers, but challenges remain in ensuring equitable access to medical care. Heavy patient loads, an aging population with comorbidities, and healthcare staffing shortages create a high-risk environment for errors. A CDC report (2011) found that the majority of ED visits involve urgent or emergent cases, reinforcing the essential role of EDs despite systemic pressures.

Legal Considerations and Professional Liability

Legal risks in the ED include both general liability and professional liability. General liability encompasses issues such as environmental hazards, while professional liability focuses on allegations of negligence or omissions in patient care. Negligence claims require the presence of four elements:

1. Duty of care owed to the patient.

2. Breach of that duty.

3. Resultant patient injury or damages.

4. Direct causation between the breach and harm.

Malpractice lawsuits can significantly impact nursing professionals. Although only 5% of claims proceed to trial, nurses remain vulnerable to litigation. Preparation, awareness, and adherence to protocols can mitigate these risks.

The Litigation Process: Anatomy of a Lawsuit

When a malpractice claim arises, the process typically unfolds in distinct stages:

1. Notification: The defendant receives a Summons and Complaint.

2. Discovery: Both parties collect evidence, including medical records, deposition testimony, and policy documents.

3. Summary Judgment: A judge evaluates undisputed facts to determine whether a trial is necessary.

4. Settlement Negotiation: Attorneys may agree on a financial settlement to avoid trial.

5. Trial: If unresolved, the case proceeds to court, where a judge or jury renders a verdict.

Appeals may extend the process for years. Nurses should engage legal counsel, notify risk management, and avoid making personal promises during claims.

Professional Liability Insurance: A Detailed Overview

Coverage Provided by Employers

Healthcare facilities typically extend professional liability insurance to licensed staff during their employment. This coverage applies as long as the employee works within their scope of practice and refrains from engaging in criminal acts. However, individual healthcare professionals often wonder if additional personal liability insurance is necessary. While employer-provided policies are generally sufficient, personal coverage can be advantageous in specific scenarios:

1. Independent Representation: In cases where the employer's insurer might settle claims against your preferences or if a conflict of interest arises, having personal coverage ensures independent legal representation.

2. Regulatory Investigations: Many employer policies may not cover legal expenses for

investigations by licensing boards or regulatory agencies, making personal coverage beneficial.

Volunteer Scenarios

Employer-provided liability coverage typically extends to volunteering at hospital-sponsored events. However, for activities outside hospital scope—such as providing medical care at community events or sports games—healthcare professionals must confirm whether the hosting organization offers liability insurance for potential claims.

Good Samaritan Laws

Emergent situations encountered off duty may compel healthcare professionals to assist. While fear of litigation is common, Good Samaritan laws in most states protect rescuers, provided they act without expectation of compensation and avoid gross negligence.

These laws vary by state, with some offering protection only to trained medical personnel or specific interventions like CPR or hemorrhage control.

Healthcare providers must familiarize themselves with their state-specific Good Samaritan statutes.

## Coping with Litigation Stress: Support for the "Second Victim"

Being named in a lawsuit can be emotionally taxing, leading to isolation, workplace tension, and significant stress. Individuals involved, directly or indirectly, are often termed "second victims." Common triggers include witnessing an incident, documenting care, or being involved in the patient's care during the event.

Symptoms of Stress Among Second Victims:

Emotional distress (e.g., guilt, anger, frustration)

Sleep disturbances and fatigue

Difficulty concentrating

Physical symptoms such as tremors or elevated blood pressure


Strategies to Mitigate Stress:

Engage in social activities and share experiences with trusted individuals.

Maintain a healthy lifestyle through regular exercise, adequate rest, and balanced nutrition.

Seek professional counseling when needed.

Avoid self-medicating or relying on alcohol.


Common Litigation Allegations in Emergency Medicine

Understanding frequent causes of malpractice claims allows healthcare providers to adopt proactive, evidence-based strategies to prevent similar occurrences. According to a report by the Physician Insurers Association of America (PIAA), diagnostic errors account for 49% of emergency department malpractice claims, with other significant contributors being procedural errors and medication-related mistakes.

Frequent Allegations Include:

Failure to Diagnose: Conditions such as myocardial infarction, appendicitis, or meningitis.

Improper Procedural Performance: Inadequate patient assessment or physical exams.

Medication Errors: Incorrect dosage, drug omissions, or administering the wrong medication.

Standards of Care in Nursing Practice

Healthcare professionals have a legal obligation to provide care aligning with established standards. These standards are determined by factors such as:

1. Community Standards: Comparing a provider's actions to those of peers in similar settings.

2. State-wide Standards: Avoiding discrepancies between small and larger community practices.

3. National Standards: Defined by regulatory agencies and case law precedents.

Maintaining up-to-date knowledge of standards through continuing education and familiarity with institutional policies is critical. Hospital policies and procedures, often reviewed during legal proceedings, must remain current to reflect the best practices.

Role of Regulatory Bodies

Federal and state regulatory agencies enforce compliance through statutes and regulations. Examples include:

1. Centers for Medicare & Medicaid Services (CMS): Ensures quality, cost-effective care by auditing medical necessity, patient experience, and treatment efficacy.

2. Centers for Disease Control and Prevention (CDC): Monitors infectious diseases, requiring mandatory reporting and providing guidelines for prevention and control.

3. Food and Drug Administration (FDA): Regulates the safety and efficacy of medications, devices, and clinical trials.

4. Occupational Safety and Health Administration (OSHA): Oversees workplace

safety, particularly regarding hazardous materials and workplace injuries.

Accreditation Agencies

Accreditation organizations, such as The Joint Commission (TJC), DNV-GL, and HFAP, play a pivotal role in maintaining standards of care. These entities evaluate healthcare facilities for compliance with CMS requirements and employ quality indicators to enhance performance.

Risk Identification: Enhancing Patient Safety and Mitigating Harm

Risk identification is a critical component in advancing patient safety and minimizing harm within healthcare systems. Delivering care occurs in a dynamic and complex environment characterized by rapid advancements in technologies and treatment modalities. This constant evolution challenges nurse educators and departmental leaders to maintain the proficiency and education of their teams. Risks may be identified through various sources, including patients, visitors, clinical and non-clinical staff, and external vendors. Ideally, risk identification should be proactive, allowing for the implementation of strategies to address potential vulnerabilities before they result in adverse outcomes. Reactive identification, though necessary in some cases, is suboptimal as it signifies that harm has already occurred.

Proactive Risk Identification Approaches

Proactive measures to identify and mitigate risks are essential, although, in practice, they are often implemented only after a negative outcome. Retrospective analyses of adverse events expose system weaknesses, providing the basis for corrective actions to prevent recurrence. However, the ideal approach involves identifying risks before incidents occur. Several methodologies have been developed to support proactive risk assessment in healthcare.

Failure Mode and Effects Analysis (FMEA)

Initially developed by engineers for evaluating military systems, Failure Mode and Effects Analysis (FMEA) has been adapted by the healthcare industry to systematically identify process vulnerabilities and their potential impact. This method aids in prioritizing improvement initiatives and involves the following steps:

1. Mapping out all steps within a process.

2. Identifying potential failures at each step.

3. Analyzing the root causes of these failures.

4. Assessing the consequences of each failure.

Each aspect is assigned a score, which determines the overall risk level associated with the failure. Prioritized risks are then addressed through targeted interventions to prevent recurrence. For example, if a nurse inadvertently administers 50 mg of a medication instead of the prescribed 25 mg and the error is later adjusted by the physician, this incident remains a reportable medication error.

Event Reporting: Capturing Near Misses and Good Catches

Reporting adverse events, near misses, and "good catches" is vital for understanding organizational vulnerabilities and improving patient safety processes. These reports inform leadership about error trends, highlight processes needing improvement, and may alert risk managers to potential legal issues or mandatory disclosure obligations. However, underreporting remains a challenge, often stemming from fear of disciplinary action or cumbersome reporting procedures.

A culture of safety, where errors are viewed as opportunities for system improvement rather than individual fault, encourages transparent reporting. Institutions fostering such cultures often report higher volumes of events, including near misses. Leadership must demonstrate trustworthiness and ensure follow-up actions to reassure staff that their concerns are being addressed.

Reactive Approaches to Risk Management

Despite the benefits of proactive risk identification, healthcare organizations often rely on reactive strategies. These strategies involve investigating adverse events after they occur to understand their root causes and implement preventive measures.

Sentinel Events and Root Cause Analysis (RCA)

Sentinel events—unexpected occurrences involving death or serious injury—prompt immediate action to prevent recurrence.

Conducting a Root Cause Analysis (RCA) involves the following steps:

1. Documenting the processes leading to the event.

2. Comparing actual processes with established policies or protocols.

3. Identifying deviations or workarounds and understanding why they occurred.

4. Evaluating process, human, and environmental factors to develop a comprehensive action plan.

For example, a medication error might be traced to a nurse retrieving the wrong drug from a dispensing machine. While initial solutions might focus on educating the nurse, further investigation could reveal that the machine's slots were incorrectly stocked. Addressing the root stocking issue ensures long-term prevention.

The Role of Transparency and Self-Reporting

The Joint Commission encourages healthcare organizations to self-report sentinel events to facilitate trend analysis and global knowledge-sharing. While concerns about litigation may discourage reporting, transparency allows institutions to access quality improvement tools, such as Sentinel Event Alerts and annual root cause trend reports. These resources support the development of targeted risk management and patient safety plans.

Mandatory Reporting and Legal Obligations

Federal and state laws mandate reporting specific conditions, such as firearm injuries or abuse cases, to ensure public health and safety. Compliance with mandatory reporting requirements is authorized under the Health Insurance Portability and Accountability Act (HIPAA), which permits the disclosure of personal health information for public health purposes, treatment coordination, and quality improvement activities.

Duty to Warn Third Parties

Healthcare providers may have a duty to warn individuals of potential harm, including notifying exposed individuals of infectious diseases or advising patients about medication-related risks. For instance, states often require physicians to report communicable diseases to public health authorities to facilitate contact tracing and mitigate outbreaks. Similarly, providers must warn patients about the risks associated with certain medications, such as avoiding heavy machinery while using sedatives.

Conclusion: Building a Robust Risk Management Framework

Effective risk management in healthcare combines proactive and reactive strategies. Facilities must prioritize proactive risk identification tools like FMEA while maintaining robust reactive measures such as RCA for addressing sentinel events. A transparent, safety-focused culture that encourages event reporting and compliance with legal obligations is fundamental to minimizing risks and enhancing patient safety.

Primary Causes of Unexpected Events in Healthcare

Healthcare involves complex interactions among numerous professionals and systems, each contributing to patient care. Even for a seemingly straightforward procedure, such as obtaining a chest X-ray, a chain of coordinated actions is required. Typically, a physician initiates the order, followed by administrative processing by unit secretaries and radiology staff. Nurses prepare patients for transport, radiology technicians perform the imaging, and radiologists interpret the results. Additionally, behind-the-scenes contributors such as biomedical engineers, housekeeping staff, and IT personnel ensure seamless operation of equipment, facility maintenance, and system functionality.

However, the intricacy of these processes makes healthcare systems vulnerable to failures. Such inadequacies can lead to unanticipated outcomes. A thorough understanding of these systems is crucial for mitigating risks and improving patient safety.

Process Failures

The Institute of Medicine's To Err Is Human: Building a Safer Health System emphasizes that most medical errors stem not from individual negligence but from systemic issues, such as faulty processes or inadequate safeguards. These errors often arise from factors such as communication breakdowns, lack of information access, or human error (Kohn et al., 2000).

For instance, a significant process failure is the neglect of follow-up for diagnostic discrepancies. A 2014 CRICO Strategies report highlighted that diagnostic errors accounted for 16% of malpractice claims in emergency departments (Hoffman, 2014). An estimated 1 in every 1,000 diagnostic encounters in outpatient settings results in harm, with approximately 5–10 patient deaths annually per average hospital due to such errors (Graber, 2014). Common contributing factors include:

Failure to address discrepancies between preliminary and final diagnostic readings.

Ineffective communication of pending test results during patient handoffs.

Inadequate policies outlining responsibilities for tracking and communicating critical results.

For example, test results returned after an emergency department (ED) admission may go unreviewed if ED staff assume inpatient teams have assumed responsibility, leading to potential oversights. Clear delegation of responsibilities and robust handoff protocols are vital to mitigate these risks.

Human Factors

Human error is a major contributor to unexpected events in healthcare, often categorized into latent conditions (systemic flaws) and active failures (individual actions). James Reason's seminal work outlines three types of active failures:

1. Slips: Unintentional actions, such as picking up the wrong medication by mistake.

2. Lapses: Omissions due to forgetfulness, like failing to follow up on test results.

3. Mistakes: Incorrect actions taken under the belief they are correct, such as administering a medication without proper authorization.

These errors differ from violations, which involve intentional deviations from standard practices (Carayon & Wood, 2010). Examples of violations include disregarding double-check protocols for high-risk medications or silencing clinical alarms.

## Script Concordance and Cognitive Bias

Clinical decision-making involves synthesizing patient data to form working diagnoses and refining them with additional information. In fast-paced environments like the ED, clinicians often rely on "scripts"—mental shortcuts formed through pattern recognition and experience. While expedient, scripts carry inherent risks of cognitive bias (Lubarsky et al., 2013).

## Common Cognitive Biases in Healthcare

1. Triage Cueing: Occurs when early diagnostic impressions unduly influence subsequent decisions. For example, documenting a patient's chief complaint in subjective terms ("constipation") rather than objective descriptions may lead to underestimating severity.

2. Visceral Bias: Emotional responses, either positive or negative, can skew clinical judgment. Negative labeling of patients, such as referring to them as "frequent flyers," risks overlooking serious conditions, such as epidural abscess in chronic pain patients.

3. Anchoring Bias: Fixating on an initial diagnosis despite conflicting evidence. For instance, attributing fatigue, shortness of breath, and abnormal vital signs to anxiety might delay diagnosis and treatment of a myocardial infarction.

4. Confirmation Bias: Seeking evidence to confirm rather than challenge an initial hypothesis. For example, interpreting diminished breath sounds as a minor issue without exploring alternative explanations may lead to missed diagnoses.

Awareness and mitigation of these biases are essential for accurate diagnosis and treatment. Strategies include comprehensive documentation, fostering open communication, and employing systematic approaches to patient assessment.

Effective Team Communication

Effective communication is a cornerstone of high-performing teams, particularly in high-stress environments such as emergency departments (ED). To maintain effective communication during periods of chaos, leaders must establish a shared understanding of the team's purpose and ensure alignment on objectives. Tasks should be delegated explicitly to specific team members rather than relying on general verbal commands. Clear delegation minimizes ambiguity and ensures accountability. Additionally, fostering an environment where all team members, regardless of hierarchy, feel empowered to voice concerns about patient safety or adverse conditions is crucial for optimal outcomes.

Documentation in Healthcare

Accurate and timely documentation is integral to ensuring continuity of care among healthcare providers. In the ED, where workflows can become overwhelmed, there is an increased risk of delayed or incomplete documentation. This delay can lead to inaccuracies in capturing critical events such as procedures performed, medications administered, and patient responses. Furthermore, during busy shifts, there is a heightened likelihood of documentation errors, such as entering data into the wrong patient's record. To mitigate these risks, providers should prioritize reviewing and updating patient records during or before the end of their shift, ensuring the accuracy and completeness of medical records.

Aftercare Instructions

Providing clear aftercare instructions is vital to extending care beyond the ED visit and preventing potential complications. Patients' understanding of these instructions can significantly impact their recovery trajectory. However, numerous factors can impede comprehension, including pain, fatigue, language barriers, literacy challenges, or the effects of acute stress.

Evidence suggests that ED patients forget up to 80% of discharge instructions by the time they leave the premises. To counteract this, healthcare teams should:

Provide legible, printed instructions tailored to the patient's condition.

Use large fonts for patients with visual impairments and ensure the language used is comprehensible to individuals with lower literacy levels.

Offer interpreter services for non-English-speaking patients, as studies have shown family members may misinterpret up to 52% of critical information.

Highlight critical information and explicitly invite patients to return to the ED if their condition worsens.

Providers should avoid asking general questions like, "Do you have any questions?" and instead confirm understanding by asking, "What is your understanding of when to return to the ED?"

Risk Mitigation Strategies

Proactively identifying and addressing potential risks is essential to delivering quality care. Effective risk mitigation involves devising strategies to minimize adverse outcomes. Examples include enhanced monitoring for high-risk conditions, adherence to clinical guidelines, and fostering a culture of safety awareness.

Continuous Quality Improvement

Improving the quality of care is an ongoing endeavor that requires the systematic identification of clinical challenges, evidence-based solutions, and the integration of new practices. Hospitals often rely on internal quality improvement committees and external benchmarks, such as those set by the Centers for Medicare & Medicaid Services (CMS) and The Joint Commission.

In 2001, the Institute of Medicine (IOM) emphasized six core aims for healthcare: safe, effective, patient-centered, timely, efficient, and equitable care. Building on these principles, the Institute for Healthcare Improvement (IHI) launched the Triple Aim initiative in 2007, focusing on enhancing patient experience, improving population health, and reducing costs.

Core and Accountability Measures

Core measures, originally established by The Joint Commission, track the quality of care for specific high-risk conditions like pneumonia and heart failure. These evidence-based metrics aim to enhance timeliness and effectiveness in care delivery. To ensure reliability, accountability measures were introduced in 2011, requiring adherence to strict criteria, including:

Scientific Evidence: Demonstrating improved outcomes through the intervention.

Proximity: Direct correlation between the measure and patient outcomes.

Accuracy: Precise evaluation of process adherence.

Safety: Minimal risk of adverse effects.

Preventing Never Events

Never events—serious, preventable errors such as wrong-site surgeries or hospital-acquired infections—are rare but devastating. CMS has ceased reimbursement for many such incidents, emphasizing their prevention. Conversely, the IHI's events always focus on positive practices, such as respectful communication, thorough hand hygiene, and bedside handoffs that include the patient in the care plan.

Clinical Practice Guidelines

Clinical practice guidelines serve as a bridge between research and practical application. These evidence-based recommendations guide healthcare providers in addressing complex clinical issues, including patient throughput, alarm management, and reducing risks for boarded patients. By regularly updating guidelines based on new research, institutions ensure that care remains aligned with the highest standards.

Regulatory Compliance

Federal regulations, such as the Emergency Medical Treatment and Active Labor Act (EMTALA) and the Health Insurance Portability and Accountability Act (HIPAA), profoundly influence ED operations. EMTALA mandates care for all individuals regardless of ability to pay, while HIPAA safeguards patient privacy and facilitates secure information sharing. Compliance with these laws ensures that care delivery is equitable and respectful of patient rights.

Overview of EMTALA Requirements

Compliance with the Emergency Medical Treatment and Labor Act (EMTALA) is fundamental in emergency care. When a patient arrives at the Emergency Department (ED) seeking medical evaluation, they are first triaged based on the severity of their condition. Subsequently, a qualified medical provider (QMP) conducts a medical screening examination (MSE) to identify if the patient has an emergency medical condition (EMC). This evaluation may range from a simple assessment (e.g., examining a rash) to more complex processes, including diagnostic imaging, laboratory tests, and consultations. Importantly, the same level of care must be provided to all patients, irrespective of their insurance status or ability to pay. Any deviation from this standard may result in investigations or penalties under EMTALA.

If an EMC is identified, stabilization is the immediate priority using all available resources within the facility. Should the patient require advanced care beyond the facility's capabilities, a transfer to a higher-level care center must be arranged. Once the EMC is either ruled out or stabilized, EMTALA obligations cease, and the patient may be discharged or transferred for follow-up care.

Core Principles of EMTALA

1. Equal Treatment: Patients must receive necessary evaluations and interventions without regard to their financial or insurance status.

2. Stabilization Priority: Every effort must be made to stabilize the patient before discharge or transfer.

3. Safe Transfers: If transfer is necessary, it must be to a facility with adequate resources to manage the patient's condition. The transfer

must also comply with specific documentation and consent requirements.

## Capacity and Capability

A hospital's capacity is determined not only by its stated resources but also by its ability to exceed those limits during emergencies. For instance, if a hospital with a capacity of 200 beds routinely accommodates up to 205 patients, the latter figure is considered its effective capacity under EMTALA.

## Distinction Between Triage and MSE

It is critical to distinguish triage from an MSE. Triage involves prioritizing patients based on acuity but does not constitute a comprehensive medical evaluation. Only QMPs, as defined by the hospital's rules and regulations, may perform an MSE. While emergency physicians are typically qualified for MSEs, other providers, such as perinatal nurses, may only conduct limited evaluations, such as ruling out labor in pregnant patients, provided they adhere to their defined scope of practice.

Risks of Noncompliance

Delays in performing an MSE or failure to follow EMTALA protocols can expose hospitals and providers to significant legal and financial penalties. Common compliance issues include:

Delayed MSEs or stabilization efforts.

Failure to provide ongoing care throughout the ED stay.

Improper documentation of reasons, risks, and benefits during patient transfers.

Non-response from on-call physicians.

Patient Transfers

Under EMTALA, transfers are permissible only for two reasons:

1. Patient Request: The patient or their representative explicitly requests the transfer after understanding its risks and benefits.

2. Higher-Level Care: The patient requires advanced care unavailable at the current facility to stabilize their EMC.

Key steps in arranging a transfer include:

Explaining the reasons, risks, and benefits of the transfer in clear terms.

Documenting the patient's consent thoroughly.

Certifying the patient's stability for transfer.

Ensuring appropriate transportation arrangements, including qualified personnel and necessary equipment.

Reporting Violations

Hospitals are required to report suspected EMTALA violations within 72 hours. Examples of reportable offenses include transferring patients without prior acceptance from the receiving facility or withholding care due to insurance issues.

Documentation and Best Practices

Proper documentation is crucial for EMTALA compliance. Utilizing checklists can help ensure completeness but does not guarantee accuracy. Key elements include:

Names, dates, and times of accepting providers.

Comprehensive documentation of consent discussions and clinical assessments.

Immediate transport even if some documentation is incomplete, with a note indicating follow-up.

Interfacing with HIPAA

Compliance with the Health Insurance Portability and Accountability Act (HIPAA) is equally important. HIPAA safeguards protected health information (PHI), including demographic data and medical diagnoses. Any breaches, even inadvertent, can result in significant fines, particularly when stemming from willful neglect.

Implementing Best Practices in Healthcare

The concept of best practices in healthcare revolves around adopting effective, proven strategies that improve patient outcomes while reducing risks. By sharing successful practices among hospitals, the healthcare community can avoid duplicating efforts and wasting resources. This section explores several best practices currently used in the healthcare industry.

Staffing Ratios in the Emergency Department

There has long been a belief that appropriate nurse staffing ratios directly impact patient outcomes. In 2004, California led the way by passing legislation mandating minimum nurse-to-patient ratios in hospitals, especially in high-acuity areas. This law aimed to standardize nurse staffing based on patient acuities, although it did not necessarily account for real-time patient needs. Following California's lead, Congress enacted the Registered Nurse Safe Staffing Act in 2013, requiring hospitals receiving Medicare to establish nurse staffing committees to tailor staffing plans according to the unique needs of their patients.

Although several states now regulate nurse staffing ratios, California remains the only one that mandates fixed staffing levels at all times. For example, in the emergency department (ED), a minimum of two nurses must be present at all times. However, studies evaluating the effectiveness of these staffing ratios have shown mixed results. A study conducted in California compared ED performance before and after the implementation of mandatory staffing ratios. The results indicated that while staffing levels increased, the time from registration to treatment and discharge also grew. Despite these changes, quality indicators, such as medication errors and patient care outcomes, showed minimal improvements.

Other research has focused on the composition of the nursing staff, emphasizing the importance of education and experience (staff mix) over sheer numbers. This aligns with the Emergency Nurses Association's position on staffing and productivity, highlighting that an optimal staffing model requires continuous evaluation through research to ensure effective patient care outcomes.

Risk Assessments

In the emergency setting, early identification of high-risk conditions is crucial. Risk assessments, often incorporated into electronic medical records (EMRs), help identify potential risks like falls and suicides. These assessments are effective only when acted upon. For instance, identifying fall risks early in the ED can prevent further complications, especially for elderly patients, who are particularly vulnerable. The use of specific fall-risk tools, which account for physiological factors like alcohol intoxication, altered mental states, and other health issues, is critical in the ED setting.

Suicide risk assessments are also vital in identifying patients at risk of self-harm. Given that 10% of suicides occur within two months of an ED visit, it is essential for providers to conduct thorough evaluations of suicidal ideation and elopement risks. Identifying these patients early and ensuring proper monitoring can save lives.

Evidence-Based Protocols

Evidence-based protocols are increasingly utilized to guide the treatment of acute conditions like ST-segment elevation myocardial infarction (STEMI), stroke, and sepsis in the ED. These protocols help healthcare providers respond quickly to life-threatening conditions by offering a standardized approach based on the latest research. While initial concerns over these protocols, such as the potential to lead to overly standardized care, have been raised, the evidence now supports their role in improving patient outcomes, including reducing morbidity and mortality.

Simulation in Medical Training

Simulation-based training allows healthcare providers to practice low-frequency, high-acuity scenarios in a controlled, risk-free environment. This technique fosters competency and confidence in handling emergency situations. Simulation can range from simple tasks, such as administering injections, to complex procedures using high-fidelity mannequins and computers.

By engaging in simulations, healthcare providers can enhance their skills, improve team communication, and build muscle memory for real-life emergencies.

Documentation Practices

Accurate and thorough documentation is critical for patient care, legal compliance, and communication between healthcare providers. It ensures continuity of care, supports billing, and serves as evidence in case of litigation. In the ED, documentation provides a clear timeline of the patient's condition, treatments, and responses. However, it can be time-consuming, with studies showing that documentation mandates add significant time to patient care. While many EDs have transitioned to electronic medical records (EMRs), paper records are still in use in some settings.

Paper Records: Despite the shift toward digital, some hospitals continue to use hybrid systems where paper records are scanned into the EMR.

Paper records can be quickly accessed, offer a more personal touch in communication, and facilitate contemporaneous documentation. However, they have drawbacks, including legibility issues, the risk of misfiled or lost pages, and challenges in meeting regulatory compliance.

Electronic Medical Records (EMRs): EMRs are increasingly the standard in EDs. They offer several advantages, including easier access to patient information, legible entries, and integration of alerts for high-risk assessments and protocols (e.g., for sepsis or stroke). However, EMRs may not always be tailored for the specific needs of EDs, and there can be issues with system integration across different departments or hospitals. Despite these challenges, EMRs remain a key tool for improving efficiency and patient care in the ED.

Minimum Documentation Standards

Minimum documentation standards are established by the Centers for Medicare & Medicaid Services (CMS), state regulations, accreditation bodies, professional organizations, and hospital policies. Adherence to CMS requirements is crucial, as it directly impacts Medicare reimbursement. The CMS Conditions of Participation, specifically §482.24(c), outlines the essential components of medical records. These must include information to justify admission, support the diagnosis, and document the patient's progress and response to treatments and medications (CMS, 1986).

Key Principles of Documentation

Accurate and comprehensive documentation is essential. Document all key communications within the medical record, specifying the method of communication, the participants involved, the facts presented, the recommendations given, and the decisions made. The following guidelines emphasize the necessary components of proper documentation and the behaviors to avoid.

Documentation Guidelines

Always Include:

Serial assessments focused on the presenting complaint.

Acknowledgment and clarification of discrepancies.

Addressing abnormal vital signs.

Objective observations (e.g., "Patient reports pain level of 7/10").

Documentation of patient response to treatments and medications, along with subsequent actions.

Changes in condition, if applicable.

Accurate timestamp if documenting at a later time.

Avoid:

Subjective statements like "pain improved."

Using the "copy/paste" function in the electronic medical record (EMR).

Keeping personal copies of shift notes.

Adding addendums after the patient's departure.

Multiple open records at once.

Using default EMR settings like "normal" or "within normal limits" without further clarification.

Legal Risks for Emergency Department Nurses

The emergency department (ED) environment presents several risks for both patients and healthcare providers, including legal and physical hazards. While some risks are intrinsic to the job, others may arise unexpectedly. Being aware of and mitigating these risks is crucial to reducing legal exposure for ED nurses.

Informed Consent

In the landmark case Schloendorff v. Society of New York Hospital (1914), the court affirmed that every competent adult has the right to make decisions regarding their own body, and performing medical procedures without consent constitutes assault. Failure to obtain informed consent or exceeding the scope of consent can lead to legal consequences.

There are four main types of consent:

1. Consent for Services: Typically included in the Conditions of Admission form, granting permission for procedures such as examinations, lab tests, sutures, or X-rays.

2. Implied Consent: Assumed in emergency situations where a patient is unconscious and would reasonably consent to treatment if able. The definition of an emergency may vary by state.

3. Informed Consent: A process involving a discussion between the healthcare provider and patient, where the risks, benefits, and alternatives of a procedure are explained. This process must be documented, including the procedure's name, the practitioner performing it, and the patient's understanding of the associated risks and benefits.

4. Informed Refusal: When a patient refuses treatment, a similar process of informed discussion should be documented, with an effort to understand the reasons behind the refusal.

The healthcare provider should ensure that patients fully understand the procedure, and document their understanding in the medical record.

## Impact of the Affordable Care Act (ACA)

The Affordable Care Act (ACA), effective January 1, 2014, mandates healthcare coverage for all individuals. Its goals include improving access to healthcare, expanding insurance coverage, implementing payment reforms, and enhancing quality reporting. While the ACA encourages patients to consult their primary care provider before visiting the ED, early reports show that the majority of patients continue to present at the ED. According to a survey by the American College of Emergency Physicians (2015), 75% of respondents indicated an increase in ED patient volumes since the ACA's implementation, with physicians spending more time coordinating follow-up care. This increased volume poses challenges to ED efficiency and patient satisfaction.

## The Role of Telemedicine in the ED

Telemedicine holds promise in the ED by facilitating consultations with specialists remotely, improving patient flow, and expediting care during peak times. Hospitals have used tele-radiology and tele-psychiatry for years, and now, remote emergency physicians are being explored to assist in managing busy EDs. However, using telemedicine requires patient consent and the presence of a healthcare provider during the remote examination. While telemedicine is still evolving, it offers potential for enhancing care quality and timeliness, though the legal implications of liability exposure remain uncertain.

The Use of Scribes in the ED

Scribes are unlicensed physician extenders employed in many EDs to assist with documentation and clerical tasks. They work under the direct supervision of an emergency physician and help with documenting patient history, medications, allergies, and gathering test results. However, their role is strictly limited, and they are prohibited from performing certain tasks, such as:

Conducting patient interviews independently.

Relaying verbal orders to licensed personnel.

Documenting lab or radiology results.

Providing direct patient care or discharge instructions.

Electronic Communication in Healthcare

The use of electronic devices such as smartphones and tablets is increasingly common in healthcare, particularly in EDs. However, these devices present risks, such as distraction and the potential for breaches of confidentiality. E-communications, including texting and email, must be carefully managed to comply with HIPAA regulations. Clinical information should be directed to the EMR, and personal devices must be encrypted to prevent unauthorized access.

## Conclusion

The dynamic environment of the ED creates unavoidable risks to patient safety, many of which healthcare providers have limited control over, such as patient volume and the timing of arrivals. However, understanding the regulatory frameworks, being aware of legal risks, and following established guidelines can significantly improve patient safety and care quality. By using available resources to address these challenges, healthcare providers can offer safe, effective, and compassionate care, which in turn enhances both patient outcomes and job satisfaction.

## References

1. 45 CFR §164.506. (n.d.). Federal Register. Retrieved from

http://www.ecfr.gov/cgi-bin/text-idx?SID=fba47e77f90ace599e46ee1451201529&mc=true&node=se45.1.164_1506&rgn=div8

2. American College of Emergency Physicians. (2015). 2015 ACEP poll affordable care act research results. Alexandria, VA: Marketing General Incorporated.

3. American College of Emergency Physicians, American Geriatrics Society, Emergency Nurses Association, Society for Academic Emergency Medicine, & Geriatric Emergency Department Guidelines Task Force. (2014). Geriatric emergency department guidelines. Annals of Emergency Medicine, 63(5), e7–e25. https://doi.org/10.1016/j.annemergmed.2014.02.008

4. American College of Emergency Physicians. (2013). The Uninsured: Access to Medical Care Fact Sheet.

Retrieved from http://newsroom.acep.org/index.php?s=20301&item=30032

5. American Hospital Association. (2015). Always there, ready to care: The 24/7 role of America's hospitals. Chicago, IL: American Hospital Association.

6. American Nurses Association. (2014). Nurse staffing plans & ratios. Retrieved from http://www.nursingworld.org/MainMenuCategories/Policy-Advocacy/State/Legislative-Agenda-Reports/State-StaffingPlansRatios

7. Bagley, S. C. (2013). Identifying patients at risk for suicide: A brief review. Making Healthcare Safer II: An Updated Critical Analysis of the Evidence for Patient Safety Practices. Rockville, MD: Agency for Healthcare Research and Quality.

8. Brenner, I. R. (2010). How to survive a medical malpractice lawsuit: The physician's roadmap for success. San Francisco, CA: John Wiley & Sons.

9. Buckley, J. (2014). The real cost of caring or not caring. Journal of Emergency Nursing, 40(1), 68–70.

10. California Health and Safety Code 1799.102; 16 Del. C. §6801 (a); Ariz. Rev. Stat. §9-500.02; 210 ILCS 50/3.150; Minn. Stat. § 604A.01. (n.d.). Retrieved from http://www.leginfo.ca.gov/cgi-bin/displaycode?section=hsc&group=01001-02000&file=1799.100-1799.112

11. Campbell, S. G., Croskerry, P., & Bond, W. (2007). Profiles in patient safety: A "perfect storm" in the emergency department. Academic Emergency Medicine, 14(8), 743–749.

12. Carayon, P., & Wood, K. E. (2010). Patient safety: The role of human factors and systems engineering. Studies in Health Technology and Informatics, 153, 23–46.

13. Carroll, R., & Nakamura, P. B. (Eds.). (2011). Risk management handbook for healthcare organizations: The essentials (6th ed., Vol. 1, pp. 3–9, 27–32, 54–62). San Francisco, CA: John Wiley & Sons.

14. Carroll, R., & Nakamura, P. L. B. (Eds.). (2011). Risk management handbook for healthcare organizations: The essentials (6th ed., Vol. 2, pp. 8, 17–18). San Francisco, CA: John Wiley & Sons.

15. Centers for Disease Control and Prevention. (2011). National Hospital Ambulatory Medical Care Survey: 2011 Emergency Department Summary Tables. Atlanta, GA: Centers for Disease Control and Prevention.

16. Centers for Medicare & Medicaid Services. (1986). Conditions of Participation §482.24(c). Retrieved from http://www.ecfr.gov/cgi-bin/text-idx?SID=fba47e77f90ace599e46ee1451201529&mc=true&node=se42.5.482_124&rgn=div8

17. Centers for Medicare & Medicaid Services. (2014). HCAHPS: Patients' perspectives of care survey. Retrieved from http://www.cms.gov/Medicare/Quality-Initiatives-Patient-Assessment-Instruments/HospitalQualityInits/HospitalHCAHPS.html

18. Chassin, M., Loeb, J., Schmaltz, S., & Wachter, R. (2010). Accountability measures—Using measurement to promote quality improvement. New England Journal of Medicine, 363(7), 683–688.

19. Cline v. William H. Friedman & Assoc., 882 S.W. 2d 754 (Mo. Ct. App. 1994).

## Chapter 6
## Challenging Patient Populations in the Emergency Department

The emergency department (ED) is a unique microcosm, representing a cross-section of society where individuals of diverse backgrounds, socioeconomic statuses, and health conditions converge, often for urgent medical care. This environment challenges emergency nurses to provide equitable care for all patients, regardless of their personal circumstances. The ED serves as a critical safety net for people seeking medical attention, often during after-hours when other healthcare options may not be available.

Recidivism in the Emergency Department

One significant challenge is dealing with patients who frequently visit the ED, a practice referred to as recidivism. These individuals, sometimes disparagingly called "frequent flyers," often require more attention and resources due to chronic medical conditions or unmet healthcare needs. The term "frequent flyer" carries negative connotations and may foster biases among healthcare providers, ultimately affecting patient care.

Recidivism is fueled by multiple factors, including socioeconomic barriers, chronic illnesses, and inadequate access to primary care. Contrary to common misconceptions, many individuals who frequently use the ED do not fit the stereotype of being uninsured, drug-seeking, or homeless. Studies by LaCalle and Rabin (2010), and Weiss et al. (2014) found that frequent ED users often have health insurance and suffer from chronic illnesses such as cardiac diseases, renal disorders, sickle cell anemia, and legitimate pain. Moreover, a significant number of these patients also use other healthcare services, such as primary care physicians and homecare.

Despite the availability of primary care options, these patients often rely on the ED due to ineffective management of their health conditions in other settings, contributing to escalating health crises. Inadequate response to their needs in the ED can lead to worsened health conditions and feelings of neglect, further entrenching their reliance on emergency services. It is essential to avoid stigmatizing these patients and instead provide compassionate care that addresses their underlying medical issues.

Psychiatric and Behavioral Health Emergencies

Patients with psychiatric illnesses, behavioral disorders, or substance use issues are also common in the ED. The prevalence of mental health disorders in the U.S. is significant, with 8.4 million people suffering from various mental health or substance abuse conditions, including alcohol and illicit drug use (Heslin et al., 2015). Mental health issues often emerge in adolescence, with 50% of mental health disorders manifesting before the age of 14 (National Alliance on Mental Illness, 2015).

As the primary safety net for individuals with mental health and substance use disorders, the ED faces challenges in managing this complex patient group. These patients often require more time, resources, and staff attention, leading to longer ED stays that contribute to overcrowding (Stephens et al., 2014). Many EDs lack dedicated spaces for psychiatric patients, and violent behaviors—including aggression towards staff and other patients—are not uncommon. In some regions, it may take days to find an appropriate facility for transfer.

Addressing psychiatric emergencies requires a multi-faceted approach. Training emergency nurses in behavioral health management is crucial. Studies, such as those by Wolf et al. (2015), highlight that the lack of resources and specialized care often hinders effective treatment for these patients. Protocols for managing psychiatric emergencies—including the use of trained staff—can improve patient outcomes and transitions from the ED to appropriate care.

Common Psychiatric Emergencies

Patients with mental health crises may present with a wide range of conditions, including mood disorders, schizophrenia, anxiety disorders, and impulse control issues. Additionally, substance use disorders are prevalent, with patients seeking care for issues related to alcohol, opioids, cocaine, and hallucinogens.

Drug overdoses and suicidal behaviors are also common psychiatric emergencies. Prescription drug overdoses, particularly opioid painkillers and benzodiazepines, have become a significant cause of death, surpassing motor vehicle collisions in 2013 (CDC, 2015). Illicit drug use has increased, and drug-related episodes can worsen psychiatric symptoms, leading to psychotic episodes (Drug Facts, 2011).

In 2013, suicide was the tenth leading cause of death in the U.S., with firearms, hanging, and poisoning being the primary methods (American Association of Suicidality, 2015). When these patients are brought to the ED, prompt and effective intervention is critical to prevent further harm.

Initial Assessment and Management

Upon arrival, the ED nurse's first task is to assess the patient's risk for violence and ensure safety for both the patient and the staff. Factors such as male gender, drug or alcohol use, and prior violent behavior are key indicators of potential aggression (Heiner & Moore, 2014). If the patient is combative or uncooperative, healthcare providers should prioritize creating a safe environment through de-escalation strategies.

Some management techniques include:

Honesty and active listening to address the patient's concerns

Offering comfort (e.g., food, water) as appropriate

Non-confrontational communication

Screening for suicidal ideation

In more severe cases, physical restraints may be necessary, but they must be used with caution. Restraints should never be used as a means of punishment or convenience, and it is critical to ensure that restraints do not pose a medical risk to the patient. All restraints should be applied according to approved ED protocols, with careful monitoring and frequent position changes to prevent further harm.

The use of chemical restraints may also be considered in certain situations, but these should be used judiciously, in compliance with established protocols, and only when necessary to protect the patient or others from harm.

## The Homeless Patient: A Comprehensive Overview

The term "homeless" often evokes an image of an unkempt individual, perhaps holding a concealed bottle of alcohol, sitting on the street. While this portrayal is accurate for some, it is essential to recognize that homelessness is a diverse and complex issue. In January 2014, a staggering 578,424 individuals in the U.S. experienced homelessness, not necessarily living on the streets, but in cars, shelters, or makeshift dwellings (National Alliance to End Homelessness, 2015a). Many of these individuals once had stable lives, only to be pushed into homelessness by unexpected circumstances, such as job loss or a personal crisis. They often feel embarrassed, helpless, and trapped in their situation.

### Demographics of Homeless Individuals

Several key statistics provide insight into the demographic makeup of the homeless population, highlighting the complexities of their healthcare needs:

Emergency Department (ED) Utilization: 73.7% of homeless individuals admitted to the hospital entered through the ED (Karaca, Wong, & Mutter, 2013; National Health Care for the Homeless Council, 2013).

Age and Ethnicity: 16.1% of homeless patients admitted to the hospital are under 15 years old, with the racial breakdown of homeless patients in the ED being 60.2% White, 22.5% Black, and 10.6% Hispanic. Those admitted to the hospital were 19.5% White, 33.2% Black, and 15.1% Hispanic (Karaca et al., 2013; National Health Care for the Homeless Council, 2013).

Healthcare Access and Utilization

Many homeless individuals lack health insurance and financial resources, making the ED their only viable option for care. Chronic illnesses, injuries, and mental health issues often go untreated, leading to frequent ED visits, higher hospitalization rates, and longer stays compared to the general population. Some notable findings include:

Insurance Coverage: 28.1% of homeless patients admitted to the hospital are uninsured, while 42.8% of homeless patients visiting the ED are uninsured. Conversely, 48.2% of homeless individuals admitted to hospitals are covered by Medicaid (Karaca et al., 2013).

Mental Health and Substance Abuse: Among homeless patients with mental health disorders, 33.8% have schizophrenia or other psychotic disorders, and 52.8% of those treated in the ED have alcohol-related disorders (National Health Care for the Homeless Council, 2013). It is estimated that 40% of homeless individuals suffer from serious mental illnesses or chronic substance abuse disorders (National Alliance to End Homelessness, 2015b).

The Challenges of Providing Care

Homeless patients face significant barriers in receiving consistent and appropriate healthcare. They often cannot manage chronic conditions or access preventive care, which exacerbates their health issues. Simple medical interventions, such as wound dressings, can become complicated due to lack of resources and stable living conditions. For instance, homeless patients may not have a place to store medical supplies, and dressing changes may be difficult to perform without a proper setting. The situation becomes more complex if the patient requires follow-up care or hospitalization, as they may have to leave behind personal belongings or pets, which can hold deep emotional significance.

The ED is legally obligated to treat all patients, including the homeless, under the Emergency

Medical Treatment and Labor Act (EMTALA). This law ensures that hospitals with EDs must provide a medical screening examination and emergency treatment regardless of a patient's ability to pay (Centers for Medicare and Medicaid Services [CMS], 2010). However, beyond medical care, addressing the social determinants of health, such as housing and access to basic services, requires collaboration with external agencies and social workers.

The Ethical and Personal Challenges

Healthcare providers may face moral dilemmas and challenges in managing the homeless population. ED staff might develop negative attitudes, viewing these patients as "frequent flyers" seeking free services. However, it is essential to reassess these attitudes continually, ensuring that care is provided with empathy and compassion. Homeless patients endure hardships that most people cannot imagine, and they deserve the same high standard of care and attention as any other patient.

Resources and Support for the Homeless

Understanding the resources available to homeless individuals in the community is crucial for providing comprehensive care. ED staff should be familiar with local shelters, transitional housing, and services that may assist in addressing the patient's needs beyond medical treatment. This could include knowledge of shelter hours, policies on substance use, and the availability of basic necessities like showers or temporary accommodations with family members.

For more information on homelessness and resources available to this population, visit:

National Clearinghouse for Alcohol and Drug Information: samhsa.gov/nctic

Homelessness Resource Center: nrchmi.samhsa.gov

U.S. Department of Health & Human Services page for the homeless: hhs.gov/homeless

Patients with Altered Mental Status: Care Considerations

Altered mental status (AMS) is not a specific disease but a common condition in emergency departments (ED), often resulting from a range of causes, from simple hypoglycemia to more complex issues like strokes. AMS presents unique challenges for healthcare providers, especially regarding legal issues, consent, and identifying the patient's medical history. Without a known history, determining the cause of AMS and creating an effective treatment plan becomes challenging.

Understanding Mental Status

Mental status involves two main components: arousal and cognition. Arousal is controlled by the brainstem's reticular activating system, while cognition is governed by the cortical hemispheres. Conditions such as hemorrhagic strokes, head injuries, seizures, and dementia can impair these functions, leading to altered consciousness.

## Initial Management of AMS

The approach to a patient with AMS begins with the same basic principles used in other emergency cases: maintaining the airway, supporting breathing and circulation, and assessing neurological status. Immediate interventions might include:

Airway: If the patient cannot protect their airway, airway management techniques like suction, intubation, or nasopharyngeal airway placement may be necessary.

Breathing: Administer high-flow oxygen or assist ventilation if needed. In some cases, decompression of the chest or mechanical ventilation may be required.

Circulation: Monitoring pulse, blood pressure, and capillary refill to guide fluid resuscitation, control bleeding, and administer medications like vasopressors if required.

Disability: Assessing pupil reactions, neurological deficits, and potential causes of AMS (e.g., hypoglycemia or trauma).

Exposure: Removing clothing to check for underlying causes of AMS such as drug patches or signs of trauma, while minimizing heat loss.

Glasgow Coma Scale (GCS)

The Glasgow Coma Scale (GCS) is a key tool in evaluating altered mental status. It assesses eye, verbal, and motor responses, with a total score indicating the severity of the condition. Scores of 13-15 represent mild brain injury, while scores below 9 suggest a more severe impairment.

By understanding the complexities of both homeless patients and those with altered mental status, healthcare providers can deliver more effective, compassionate care tailored to the unique needs of these vulnerable populations.

Older Patients with Altered Mental Status in the Emergency Department

The Emergency Department (ED) serves as the critical point of entry for a significant number of elderly patients. In the United States, approximately 18 million individuals aged 65 and older visit the ED annually. This age group is particularly susceptible to altered mental status, including conditions such as delirium, dementia, stupor, and coma. These alterations in consciousness are not only common but can be severe and require immediate attention due to the risk of rapid deterioration and concerns for both patient and staff safety.

Stupor and coma are among the most severe forms of altered consciousness, affecting 5% to

9% of elderly patients. Prompt evaluation is crucial, as these conditions can decompensate quickly, potentially leading to life-threatening consequences. The first step in management is to identify and treat the underlying cause rather than merely addressing the symptom. For example, is the patient's condition due to a urinary tract infection (UTI), or is it a side effect of a newly prescribed medication?

One of the major challenges in emergency care for older patients is differentiating whether the change in mental status is acute or part of a chronic process. Delirium, a sudden onset alteration in mental status often due to physiological imbalances, is distinct from dementia, which develops slowly and is irreversible. However, these conditions can overlap, particularly in patients with dementia who experience delirium. The presence of delirium may obscure other treatable conditions, making accurate diagnosis critical.

Stages and Symptoms of Delirium and Dementia

Delirium is categorized into two stages (Han & Wilber, 2013; World Health Organization [WHO], 2015):

1. Hyperactive Stage:

Restlessness

Agitation

Anxiety

Combativeness

2. Hypoactive Stage:

Drowsiness

Somnolence

Lethargy

Depression

Fatigue

In some cases, patients may present with mixed symptoms of both hyperactive and hypoactive states, particularly those with dementia who develop delirium.

Dementia, on the other hand, progresses through three distinct stages:

1. Early Stage:

Forgetfulness

Disorientation to time

Getting lost in familiar places

2. Middle Stage:

Forgetting recent events and names

Difficulty with communication and self-care

Behavioral changes, including wandering and repeated questioning

3. Late Stage:

Severe disorientation, including loss of awareness of time and place

Difficulty recognizing familiar people

Increased dependence on caregivers for basic activities

Stupor and Coma

Stupor: A state of deep sleep or unresponsiveness, where the patient can only be awakened by vigorous stimulation (Han & Wilber, 2013).

Coma: A state of unresponsiveness where no stimuli can rouse the patient.

Table: Distinguishing Delirium and Dementia

| Symptom/Stages | Delirium | Dementia |
|---|---|---|
| Onset | Rapid (hours/days) | Slow (month/years) |
| Course | Waxing and waning | Progressive |
| Vital Signs/Physical Exam. | Often abnormal | Usually Normal |
| Focus | Inattention | Normal ( except in severe cases) |
| Level of | Altered | Normal |

| | | |
|---|---|---|
| consciousness | | (except in severe dementia) |
| **Cognition** | Disorganized thought | Perceptual disturbances |
| **Orientation** | Abnormal (as disease progresses) | Normal (except in severe cases) |
| **Cognitive Decline** | Reversible | Rarely reversible |
| **Sleep - Wake cycle** | Disturbed | Normal (except in severe cases) |
| **Hallucinations/Perceptual Disturbances** | May be present | Absent (except in severe cases) |
| **Cause** | Organic (e.g., Infections, Medications) | Organic (Degenerative) |

| | | |
|---|---|---|
| **Safety Risk** | Immediate | Yes. But gradual |
| **Prognosticators** | Good if treated rapidly | Poor |

Source: Han & Wilber, 2013; WHO, 2015.

Summary

Emergency department nurses play a crucial role in managing patients with altered mental status. These patients may present with a range of conditions, from psychiatric disorders to neurological emergencies, and require careful, individualized care. The complexity of managing such patients is compounded by issues such as homelessness and poverty, which often result in repeated ED visits. Nurses must be prepared to address not only the immediate health concerns but also explore resources and alternative healthcare options for patients facing long-term challenges.

The increasing frequency of psychiatric emergencies, coupled with the lack of adequate resources, places a significant burden on EDs, which are frequently the primary safety net for these patients. Long-term interventions, including social services and community-based care, are essential to addressing the root causes of these crises and supporting the overall well-being of the patients.

Alterations in mental status can stem from a wide range of conditions, making accurate diagnosis and treatment a challenge. By employing a systematic approach to assessment, diagnostics, and treatment, emergency nurses can help guide these patients toward appropriate care. The ED must not only provide urgent medical treatment but also consider the broader social and psychological needs of the patient, reflecting a holistic approach to healthcare.

Finally, the emotional and physical needs of vulnerable populations—such as the homeless and those living in poverty—must be acknowledged. For these individuals, the ED may be the only accessible healthcare resource, making compassionate care and resource referral essential to improving their overall health outcomes.

References

1. American Association of Suicidology. (2015). U.S.A. suicide: 2013 official final data. Retrieved from http://www.suicidology.org/Portals/14/docs/Resources/FactSheets/2013datapgsv3.pdf

2. Boudreaux, E., Niro, K., Sullivan, A., Rosenbaum, C., Allen, M., & Camargo, C. (2011). Current practices for mental health follow-up after psychiatric emergency department/psychiatric emergency service visits: A national survey of academic emergency departments. General Hospital Psychiatry, 31, 631–633.

3. Centers for Disease Control and Prevention (CDC). (2012). Chartbook: Special feature on emergency care. Retrieved from http://www.cdc.gov/nchs/data/hus/hus12.pdf

4. Centers for Disease Control and Prevention (CDC). (2015). Prescription drug overdose. Retrieved from http://www.cdc.gov/drugoverdose/data/overdose.html

5. Centers for Medicare and Medicaid Services (CMS). (2010). State operations manual. Retrieved from http://www.cms.gov/Regulations-and-Guidance/Guidance/Manuals/Downloads/som107ap_v_emerg.pdf

6. Christensen, B. (2014). Glasgow Coma Scale – Adult. Retrieved from http://emedicine.medscape.com/article/2172603-overview

7. Drug Facts. (2011). Addiction and other mental disorders. Retrieved from http://www.drugabuse.gov/publications/drugfacts/comorbidity-addiction-other-mental-disorders

8. Foster, S., LeFauve, C., Kresky-Wolff, M., & Richards, L. D. (2010). Services and support for individuals with co-occurring disorders and long-term homelessness. Journal of Behavioral Health Services and Research, 37(7), 239–251.

9. Han, J. H., & Wilber, S. T. (2013). Altered mental status in older emergency department patients. Clinical Geriatric Medicine, 29(1), 101–136.

10. Harris, S. N., & Pitman, J. (2014, June 10). Altitude illness: cerebral syndromes. MedScape. Retrieved from http://emedicine.medscape.com/article/768478-overview

11. Heiner, J., & Moore, J. (2014). The combative patient. In J. Marx, R. Hockberger, & R. Walls (Eds.), Rosen's emergency medicine (8th ed., pp. 2414–2421). Philadelphia, PA: Elsevier Saunders.

12. Heslin, K., Elixhauser, A., & Steiner, S. (2015). Hospitalizations involving mental and substance use disorders among adults. Rockville, MD: Agency for Healthcare Research and Quality. Retrieved from https://www.hcup-us.ahrq.gov/reports/statbriefs/sb191-Hospitalization-Mental-Substance-Use-Disorders-2012.jsp

13. Karaca, Z., Wong, H., & Mutter, R. (2013, March). Statistical brief #152: Characteristics of homeless individuals using inpatient and emergency department services, 2008. Retrieved from https://www.hcup-us.ahrq.gov/reports/statbriefs/sb152.pdf

14. LaCalle, E., & Rabin, E. (2010). Frequent users of emergency departments: The myths, the data and the policy implications. Annals of Emergency Medicine, 56(1), 42–47.

15. Montejano, A. (2015). Psychiatric emergencies. In L. Visser, A. Montejano, & V. Grossman (Eds.), Fast facts for the triage nurse (pp. 155–159). New York, NY: Springer.

16. Morrissey, T. (2013). CDEM self-study modules: The approach to altered mental status. Retrieved from http://www.cdemcurriculum.org/index.php/ssm/show_ssm/approach_to/ams

17. National Alliance on Mental Illness (NAMI). (2015). Facts on children's mental health in America. Retrieved from http://www.nami.org/Template.cfm?Section=Federal_and_State_Policy_Legislation

&template=/ContentManagement/Content Display.cfm&ContentID=43804

18. National Alliance to End Homelessness. (2015a, April 1). Executive summary. Retrieved from http://endhomelessness.org/library/entry/the-state-of-homelessness-in-america-2015

19. National Alliance to End Homelessness. (2015b, April 1). Health care. Retrieved from http://www.endhomelessness.org/pages/mental_physical_health

20. National Health Care for the Homeless Council. (2013, September). Integrated care quick guide: Integrating behavioral health & primary care in the HCH setting. Retrieved from http://www.nhchc.org/wp-content/uploads/2013/10/integrated-care-quick-guide-sept-2013.pdf

21. Stephens, R., White, S., Cudnik, M., & Patterson, E. (2014). Factors associated with longer length of stay for mental health emergency department patients. The Journal of Emergency Medicine, 47(4), 412–419.

22. Veterans Health Administration. (n.d.). Prudent layperson fact sheet. Retrieved from http://www.pugetsound.va.gov/docs/prudentlaypersonfactsheet.pdf

## Chapter 7
## The Emergency Nurse and the Abused Patient

The Reality of Abuse in Emergency Care

Daily news often highlights humanity's propensity for unkindness, which manifests through emotional disregard, harm to belongings or persons, and even physical or emotional violence leading to fatal outcomes. Tragically, emergency departments (EDs) often become the frontline for managing the consequences of this cruelty. Patients suffering from abuse, especially vulnerable groups such as children and the elderly, evoke a profound sense of empathy in healthcare providers.

Emergency nurses hold a dual responsibility—not only to treat victims of abuse but also to recognize the signs, intervene, and connect individuals with resources to escape these situations. This chapter explores various forms of abuse encountered in the ED, their manifestations, and appropriate interventions to support these victims.

Child Abuse: A Persistent Threat

Historical Context and Legislation

Child abuse has been a persistent issue, recognized as a medical and social problem warranting legislative action only in the last six decades. The Child Abuse Prevention and Treatment Act (CAPTA), enacted on January 31, 1974, and reauthorized in December 2010, sets the framework for child protection laws across the United States. CAPTA defines child abuse as:

> "Any recent act or failure to act on the part of a parent or caretaker which results in death, serious physical or emotional harm, sexual abuse or exploitation; or an act or failure to act which presents an imminent risk of serious harm."

Types of Child Abuse

Child abuse typically falls into four categories:

1. Neglect

Basic Needs: Failure to provide essentials such as food, shelter, or clothing.

Emotional Neglect: Exposing a child to domestic violence or humiliation.

Medical Neglect: Ignoring necessary healthcare, including dental care.

Educational Neglect: Failing to enroll a child in school or address special educational needs.

2. Physical Abuse

Infliction of physical harm through actions like shaking, burning, or hitting.

## 3. Sexual Abuse

Includes acts such as genital fondling, exploitation through human trafficking, and exposure to pornographic materials.

## 4. Psychological Abuse

Actions causing severe cognitive or emotional disorders.

## Mandatory Reporting

All healthcare professionals, including nurses, are legally required to report suspected child abuse to child protective services (CPS).

## Prevalence of Child Abuse

## Challenges in Assessment

Quantifying child abuse is complicated by underreporting, lack of identification, and unrecognized cases. Key studies such as the National Child Abuse and Neglect Data System (NCANDS) and National Incident Studies (NIS) provide valuable insights:

In 2013, 3.5 million referrals involving 6.4 million children were reported to CPS. Of these, 679,000 cases were confirmed, with 1,520 fatalities, 70% of which involved children under three years old.

The Centers for Disease Control and Prevention (CDC) estimates the lifetime cost of confirmed abuse cases for a single year to be $124 billion (2014).

Despite these numbers, it is believed that CPS-reported cases significantly underestimate the true prevalence. For instance, a 2013 study revealed that 1 in 4 children in the United States experiences abuse during their lifetime.

## Demographics of Abuse

### By Ethnicity

Child abuse crosses socioeconomic and cultural lines. However, data from the CDC (2014) highlights disparities among ethnic groups:

African American: 14.2%

American Indian/Alaska Native: 12.4%

Hispanic: 8.4%

Asian: 1.7%

### By Perpetrators

Parents are the most frequent perpetrators, accounting for 80.3% of reported cases. Other perpetrators include relatives (6.1%) and unmarried partners (4.2%).

Consequences of Child Abuse

The Adverse Childhood Experiences (ACE) Study, conducted by the CDC and Kaiser Permanente, links childhood abuse to long-term health risks. These include:

Chronic illnesses such as ischemic heart disease and chronic obstructive pulmonary disease.

Behavioral and social issues, including substance abuse, depression, and increased risk of intimate partner violence.

Poor quality-of-life outcomes, such as unintended pregnancies and early sexual activity.

Assessment and Identification of Child Abuse: A Comprehensive Analysis

Introduction Children presenting to the emergency department (ED) with complaints of physical abuse or neglect are uncommon. Caregivers of abused children often provide misleading or inconsistent accounts of the child's medical history and the mechanisms of injury. Nonverbal children cannot describe their experiences, and verbal children may be coerced into withholding the truth. These factors collectively complicate the identification of abuse, necessitating meticulous history-taking and comprehensive physical examination.

Comprehensive History and Examination A detailed history is essential, with questions focused on gathering the "who, what, when, where, why, and how" of the injury. Explanations provided by caregivers must align with the child's developmental abilities and the observed injuries. Discrepancies in caregivers' accounts, significant changes in explanations, or delays in seeking medical care raise suspicion. Interviews should be conducted privately, with verbal children interviewed separately when feasible. Open-ended, non-leading questions are recommended, and answers should be documented verbatim. Professional translators must be utilized when language barriers exist.

Physical Examination Protocol A thorough head-to-toe assessment is critical, ensuring the child is completely undressed and gowned. The skin, as the most commonly injured organ, should be evaluated for abrasions, contusions, lacerations, burns, bites, and patterned injuries. Specific findings that warrant concern include:

No explanation or vague accounts for significant injuries.

Inconsistent explanations with injury patterns, severity, or developmental capabilities.

Variations in witnesses' accounts.

Delays in seeking care or undisclosed past injuries.

Key Findings Indicative of Abuse

1. Bruising:

Bruises in non-cruising infants (<6 months) are highly suspicious.

Patterns of bruising inconsistent with accidental injuries, such as those on the torso, neck, or back, are concerning.

Abusive bruising may display distinct patterns, such as handprints or object imprints.

2. Burns:

Intentional burns often have clear demarcation lines or assume the pattern of objects.

Common abusive burns include "stocking" burns (feet and legs) and "doughnut" burns (buttocks submerged in hot water).

Delays in seeking care for burns further indicate intentional harm.

3. Bite Marks:

Ovoid bruises around 3 cm in diameter suggest human bite marks.

The area should be swabbed for DNA evidence before cleansing.

Differentiating Non-Abusive Conditions Medical and cultural practices must be considered to avoid misidentifying conditions as abuse. For example:

Medical conditions: Idiopathic thrombocytopenia, hemophilia, and certain dermatological disorders.

Cultural practices: Coining, cupping, and moxibustion.

Abusive Head Trauma (AHT) Abusive head trauma, a broad term encompassing injuries caused by shaking or blunt force, is a leading cause of abuse-related fatalities in children under two years. Common findings include subdural hematomas, retinal hemorrhages, skull fractures, and cervical spine injuries. The American Academy of Pediatrics advocates the use of the term "abusive head trauma" over "shaken baby syndrome" to reflect the multifaceted mechanisms of injury.

Triggers and Prevention Crying is a frequent trigger for AHT. The Period of PURPLE Crying program educates caregivers about normal infant crying patterns to prevent abuse. It emphasizes understanding that excessive crying, especially during peak periods around two months of age, is typical and temporary.

Common Triggers for Abusive Head Trauma

Skeletal Injuries

Skeletal injuries frequently occur in children, but distinguishing accidental from abusive injuries is critical. A detailed history of the injury mechanism is essential to evaluate its plausibility. Certain fracture types are more indicative of abuse than others. The table below outlined the specificity of various fractures as potential markers of inflicted trauma:

| Specificity | Signs of Abuse |
|---|---|
| **High** | Classic metaphyseal lesions (corner fracture), rib fracture (especially posterior). Scapula fracture, sternal fracture |
| **Moderate** | Multiple Fracture (; particularly bilateral), fractures in various healing stages, epiphyseal separations, vertebral body fractures/ subluxations, digital fracture, Complex skill fractures |

| Low (Most common) | Subperiosteal new bone formation, clavicle fractures, Long bone fractures, Linear skull fractures |

(Source: Kleinman, 1989, p. 9)

Abdominal Injuries

Abdominal injuries resulting from child abuse can be challenging to identify due to their delayed presentation and subtle clinical signs. Unlike accidental trauma, these injuries often lack external bruising, largely due to delayed manifestation and the lack of bony structures in the abdomen. Intentional trauma such as kicking or stomping can lead to damage to solid or hollow organs.

Clinical signs may range from mild (e.g., abdominal tenderness, rigidity, or fever) to severe (e.g., tachycardia, symptoms of hypovolemic or septic shock, and altered mental status). Abdominal trauma is rarely isolated, particularly in younger children, requiring comprehensive evaluation when suspected.

Medical Child Abuse (MCA)

The term Medical Child Abuse (MCA), formerly referred to as Munchausen Syndrome by Proxy (MSBP), describes cases where a caregiver subjects a child to unnecessary or harmful medical interventions. Symptoms may include fabricated or induced illnesses such as vomiting, apnea, or infections.

The identification of MCA requires multidisciplinary collaboration and an extensive review of the child's medical history. Children with vague symptoms or frequent emergency department visits should raise suspicion. The table below summarized common clinical presentations associated with MCA.

| Category | Clinical Findings |
|---|---|
| **Respiratory** | Apnea, Choking cyanosis, haemoptysis, respiratory abuse |
| **Cardiovascular** | Bradycardia, cardiomyopathy, shock |
| **Gastrointestinal** | Abdominal pains, feeding difficulties, vomiting, diarrhea |
| **Neurological** | Seizures, Behavioural disorders, developmental delays |
| **Skin** | Burns, abscesses rashes |

| | |
|---|---|
| **Infections** | Fever. septic arthritis, Osteomyelitis |
| **Hematological** | Easy bruising anemia |
| **Metabolic** | Electrolyte imbalances, hypoglycemia, hyperkalemia |

(Source: Rosenberg, 2009)

Interventions

Managing suspected child abuse requires a structured and systematic approach to ensure accurate diagnosis, treatment, and reporting. Key interventions include:

1. Primary Assessment

Assess airway, breathing, circulation, and neurologic status, initiating life-saving interventions as necessary.

2. Secondary Assessment

Perform a comprehensive head-to-toe examination with the child completely disrobed.

3. History Collection

Obtain a thorough medical and social history, including a detailed account of the injury mechanism.

4. Skeletal Survey

Mandatory for children under two years when abuse is suspected. Limited value exists for children aged 2–5, evaluated case-by-case.

5. Diagnostic Testing

CT Scan: Perform on the head for infants <6 months or when suspicion of cranial trauma exists.

Laboratory Tests: Include CBC, coagulation studies, liver enzymes, amylase, and lipase for suspected abdominal trauma.

Abdominal CT: Recommended if lab results or clinical evaluation suggest trauma.

Ophthalmology Consultation: Necessary for suspected head injuries to evaluate retinal hemorrhages.

6. Injury Documentation

Record injuries with photos from various perspectives (distance, mid-range, and close-up) with scale objects included. Ensure all photographs are labeled appropriately.

7. Mandatory Reporting

Notify Child Protective Services (CPS) and law enforcement.

8. Specialist Consultation

Engage child abuse specialists for guidance and case review.

9. Detailed Documentation

Maintain comprehensive notes, including verbatim quotes from caregivers and medical findings.

Skeletal Survey Guidelines

When conducting a skeletal survey, ensure all necessary views are obtained. The table below lists required components:

| Appendicular | Axial Skeleton |
| --- | --- |

| Skeleton | |
|---|---|
| Humerus (AP & lateral) | Thorax (AP & lateral) |
| Forearms (AP & lateral) | Oblique ribs |
| Hands (Oblique PA) | Pelvis ( AP with lumbar spine) |
| Femurs (AP & lateral | Cervical spine lateral |
| Lower legs (AP lateral) | Skull (frontal & lateral) |

(Source: Adapted from relevant guidelines)

Communication with Caregivers

Suspected abuse must be reported in compliance with legal obligations. It is essential to maintain transparency and open communication with caregivers, providing support to the child to mitigate emotional distress and ensure their understanding of the situation.

## Domestic Human Trafficking

### Introduction

Human trafficking represents a pervasive global health and human rights crisis, identified in over 150 countries. It encompasses sex trafficking and labor trafficking, each profoundly eroding individual dignity and humanity. Victims of sex trafficking often work in exploitative settings such as massage parlors, brothels, strip clubs, or escort services, while those subjected to labor trafficking are commonly found in roles like domestic workers, factory laborers, janitors, construction workers, and restaurant staff. Contrary to popular belief, trafficking extends beyond stereotypical urban environments, infiltrating everyday settings, which complicates detection and intervention.

Prevalence and Economic Impact

Shared Hope International's 2009 undercover investigation reveals alarming statistics: a significant number of American children are coerced into the commercial sex industry annually. Globally, human trafficking generates approximately $150 billion annually, with an estimated $9.8 billion attributed to operations within the United States alone. Domestic Minor Sex Trafficking (DMST), defined as the commercial sexual exploitation of minors under 18 years of age, disproportionately affects an estimated 100,000 children annually, with an average victim age of 13.

Forms of Trafficking and Legal Definitions

Sex Trafficking: The recruitment, harboring, or exploitation of individuals for commercial sex acts through force, fraud, or coercion. In the case of minors, any commercial sex act qualifies as trafficking regardless of consent.

Labor Trafficking: The exploitation of individuals for forced labor or services through similar means, often resulting in modern-day slavery conditions.

The commercial exchange in trafficking often involves non-monetary transactions such as food, shelter, or drugs, perpetuating cycles of control and exploitation.

Vulnerable Populations and Risk Factors

Victims often come from marginalized backgrounds, including single-parent households, foster care, or histories of abuse, neglect, or substance use. Teenage girls comprise 98% of victims, with LGBTQ+ youth and those involved with Child Protective Services (CPS) at heightened risk. Traffickers frequently exploit children in community spaces such as schools, sports events, shelters, or transportation hubs, luring them with promises of safety, employment, or love.

Common Recruitment Locations:

Schools and foster care homes

Social media platforms

Shopping malls and transit stations

Public events and shelters

Traffickers and Tactics

Traffickers, often individuals close to the victim (e.g., family members or romantic partners), manipulate children using emotional and psychological tactics. Common strategies include:

1. Grooming: Offering affection, gifts, or career opportunities to build trust.

2. Isolation and Dehumanization: Utilizing violence, threats, and blackmail, such as leveraging pornographic materials.

3. Branding: Tattooing victims with identifiable marks symbolizing ownership.

Signs of Trafficking

Healthcare providers play a critical role in identifying trafficking victims. Common indicators include:

Tattoos linked to trafficking (e.g., barcodes or names).

Signs of physical trauma, malnutrition, or psychological distress.

Accompanying individuals who dominate or control interactions.

Health Risks and Clinical Presentations

Trafficked individuals frequently present with various physical and psychological complaints, ranging from sexually transmitted infections, malnutrition, and poorly healed injuries to depression, anxiety, and post-traumatic stress disorder. Table 1 highlights these symptoms.

Identification and Reporting

Healthcare professionals are often among the few external contacts victims encounter. Recognizing subtle cues and asking specific, nonjudgmental questions can aid identification. Key inquiries include:

"Are you free to come and go as you wish?"

"Do you control your finances and identification?"

"Have you been threatened or coerced?"

When trafficking is suspected, immediate reporting to CPS or law enforcement is required. Safety protocols must prioritize the well-being of both the victim and healthcare staff.

Interventions for Trafficking Victims

Healthcare providers encountering potential trafficking victims must perform frequent evaluations of their physical, psychological, and safety needs. Effective intervention includes life-saving measures, medical treatment, and ensuring the safety of both the patient and healthcare personnel. Below is a structured approach to managing trafficking victims:

1. Primary Assessment
Initiate with life-saving measures, focusing on airway, breathing, circulation, and neurovascular status.

2. Secondary Assessment

Conduct a comprehensive head-to-toe examination. Ensure privacy while fully disrobing the patient to assess for signs of injury, untreated conditions, and nutritional deficits.

3. Medical History Collection
Document the patient's medical history, including previous treatments, medications, surgeries, and allergies.

4. Safety Measures
Involve security personnel, law enforcement, and child protective services (CPS) if necessary to safeguard both the patient and staff.

5. Initial Screening
Conduct diagnostic tests such as:

General tests: CBC, metabolic panel, toxicology, and pregnancy tests.

STI screening: HIV, RPR, gonorrhea, chlamydia, and hepatitis C tests.

Mental health evaluations: Assess for acute psychosis, suicidal ideation, and PTSD.

6. Specialist Consultation
Engage forensic or child abuse specialists for a detailed forensic examination following initial screening.

7. Comprehensive Documentation
Ensure all findings and the patient's narrative are thoroughly documented. Direct quotations should be used when noting the patient's history.

Victims often decline assistance. For adults, offer support while respecting their autonomy. Minors require mandatory notification to law enforcement and CPS. For further guidance, contact the National Trafficking Hotline at 1-888-373-7888, available 24/7 in over 200 languages.

Intimate Partner Violence (IPV)

IPV is a pervasive global health issue. The World Health Organization (WHO, 2013) highlights that 35% of women globally experience IPV, with 38% of female homicides attributed to intimate partners. Men are also victims of IPV, often facing more severe and weapon-associated violence (U.S. Department of Justice, 2013).

Emergency healthcare providers must be vigilant in identifying injuries and behaviors indicative of IPV. Non-confrontational, evidence-based screening tools promote disclosure. Statistics indicate:

Male IPV Victims: 39% face serious violence; 27% experience weapon attacks.

Female IPV Victims: More likely to receive threats or seek medical care.

Common Conditions and Complaints in IPV Patients

IPV victims often present with nonspecific symptoms or vague explanations. Common complaints include:

Psychological Symptoms: Depression, anxiety, PTSD, suicidal ideation.

Physical Complaints: Chronic pain, gastrointestinal or genitourinary symptoms, pelvic pain, unintended pregnancies, recurrent STIs, and trauma.

Communication Deficits: Cognitive issues, migraines, stroke-like symptoms, hearing or vision loss.

Screening methods should address all genders and include questions like, "Do you feel safe at home?"

LGBTQ+ and IPV

LGBTQ+ individuals face elevated IPV risks due to intersecting vulnerabilities such as race, class, and gender identity (NCAVP, 2013). Statistics reveal:

Same-sex IPV rates: 21.5% in men, 35.4% in women, compared to lower rates in opposite-sex relationships.

Providers must ensure privacy, confidentiality, and use inclusive, non-judgmental language. Referrals to LGBTQ+ support services should align with the patient's comfort regarding disclosure of sexual orientation or gender identity.

Sexual Assault

Sexual assault, as defined by the CDC, encompasses any non-consensual sexual activity, including forced penetration or acts facilitated by drugs or alcohol. Statistics show:

1 in 5 women and 1 in 69 men experience attempted or completed rape.

Risk factors include prior victimization, substance use, coercive fantasies, and societal norms tolerating sexual violence.

Patients presenting to the emergency department (ED) may seek care due to injury, fear of disease or pregnancy, or for forensic evaluation. The Violence Against Women Act (1994) established federal funding for sexual assault victims, ensuring access to forensic exams regardless of legal action. However, challenges remain in managing evidence storage and ensuring consistent follow-up care.

Emerging Issues: Youth and Digital Abuse

Adolescents and young adults increasingly face IPV through digital platforms, including sexting, cyberbullying, and electronic dating violence. Statistics show:

1 in 3 individuals aged 14–24 have sexted.

Cyberbullied youth are 3.6 times more likely to experience electronic dating violence.

Emergency care providers must assess teens comprehensively, as they are the most vulnerable to sexual assault and stalking. A structured approach ensures timely and effective intervention.

Medicolegal History and Clinical Management of Sexual Assault and Elder Abuse: Comprehensive Analysis

Medicolegal History in Sexual Assault Cases

Effective documentation and history-taking are essential in managing sexual assault cases. Key aspects of a thorough medicolegal history include the following:

1. Past Medical History:

Allergies: Identify known allergies to guide medication administration.

Medications: Record current prescriptions to avoid contraindications.

Medical/Surgical History: Understand pre-existing conditions that may influence care.

Vaccination Status: Confirm immunizations, particularly for hepatitis B.

2. Anogenital-Urinary History:

Last Consensual Intercourse: Establish a baseline for evidence comparison.

Pregnancy History: Assess risk of pregnancy and complications.

Contraceptive Use: Determine the method and efficacy of contraception.

Last Menstrual Period: Evaluate the risk of pregnancy and establish a timeline.

3. Event History:

Document the specifics of the incident, including time, location, and actions taken.

Obtain details about the assailant, use of weapons or restraints, suspected drug involvement, and physical or emotional effects.

Physical Assessment and Findings

The physical examination focuses on identifying injuries and evidence of assault. Common findings include:

General Observations: Assess demeanor, cognition, and mental status.

Clothing and Personal Items: Document torn or bloodied garments as evidence.

Injuries: Note abrasions, lacerations, bruises, petechiae, or gunshot wounds.

Anatomical Variants: Differentiate normal variants from injury-related findings.

Techniques to Enhance Evidence Collection include:

Speculum or Colposcopic Examination: For detailed visualization of injuries.

Toluidine Blue Dye Application: Highlights microabrasions.

Sterile Water Irrigation: Cleanses and reveals hidden injuries.

Comprehensive Care for Sexual Assault Victims

Care for victims is multidisciplinary, focusing on evidence collection, emotional support, and medical management. Essential interventions include:

Post-Assault Prophylaxis:

Sexually Transmitted Diseases: Administer Ceftriaxone or Cefixime combined with Azithromycin or Doxycycline.

Hepatitis B: Initiate vaccination if unvaccinated.

Pregnancy Prevention: Provide emergency contraceptives or Copper IUDs.

Follow-Up Testing: Recommend retesting for HIV and STDs at intervals of 6 weeks, 3 months, and 6 months.

Advocacy and Resources: Offer crisis center information and facilitate communication with support organizations.

Elder Abuse: Assessment and Intervention

Elder abuse encompasses physical, sexual, emotional, and financial exploitation, as well as neglect and abandonment. Key considerations include:

1. Risk Factors:

Cognitive impairments like dementia.

Dependency on caregivers.

Social isolation or financial distress.

2. Screening Questions:

"Do you feel safe where you live?"

"Has anyone ever taken your money without permission?"

"Who helps with your daily care?"

3. Physical Indicators:

General Appearance: Poor hygiene, malnutrition, or ill-fitting clothing.

Injuries: Bruises in patterns indicative of abuse, fractures, or lacerations.

Signs of Neglect: Pressure ulcers, dehydration, or untreated medical issues.

4. Sexual Abuse Indicators:

Presence of STDs or genital injuries.

Intervention Strategies:

Immediate Interventions: Stabilize life-threatening injuries and ensure patient safety.

Documentation: Photographs and detailed written descriptions of injuries.

Reporting: Notify law enforcement or Adult Protective Services as per state regulations.

Follow-Up: Coordinate referrals for medical, functional, and cognitive assessment.

Key Resources

Healthcare providers should connect patients with appropriate support systems, including:

Local rape crisis centers and elder abuse hotlines.

National organizations like the Rape, Abuse, and Incest National Network (RAINN).

Counseling services for long-term recovery from physical and emotional trauma.

## Conclusion

Proper management of sexual assault and elder abuse victims requires meticulous documentation, compassionate care, and collaboration among healthcare teams, legal authorities, and advocacy organizations. By following established protocols and leveraging available resources, providers can significantly impact patient recovery and ensure justice.

## References

1. Anglin, D., & Homeir, D. (2014). Elder abuse and neglect. In J. Marx, R. Hockberger, & R. Walls (Eds.), Rosen's Emergency Medicine (8th ed., pp. 885–892). Philadelphia, PA: Saunders.

2. Ard, K. L., & Makadon, H. L. (2011). Managing intimate partner violence among LGBTQ+ patients. Journal of General Internal Medicine, 26(8), 930–933.

3. Barr, M. (n.d.). Overview of the Period of PURPLE Crying. Retrieved from http://www.purplecrying.info

4. Basilek, K., Smith, S., Breiding, M., Black, M., & Mahendra, R. (2014). Sexual violence surveillance: Uniform definitions and recommended data elements. Retrieved from http://www.cdc.gov/violenceprevention

5. Black, A. (2012). Child maltreatment. In Emergency Nursing Pediatric Course: Provider Manual (4th ed., pp. 343–356). Des Plaines, IL: Emergency Nurses Association.

6. Black, M., Breiding, M., Smith, S., Walters, M., Merrick, M., Chen, J., & Stevens, M. (2011). The National Intimate Partner and Sexual Violence Survey: 2010 summary report. Retrieved from http://www.cdc.gov

7. Breiding, M. J., Smith, S. G., Basile, K. C., Walters, M. I., Chen, J., & Merrick, M. (2014). Prevalence and characteristics of sexual violence, stalking, and intimate partner violence in the United States, 2011. Morbidity and Mortality Weekly Report, 63(8).

8. Centers for Disease Control and Prevention (CDC). (2010). 2010 STD treatment guidelines. Retrieved from http://www.cdc.gov

9. Centers for Disease Control and Prevention (CDC). (2014a). Child maltreatment: Facts at a glance. Retrieved from www.cdc.gov

10. Centers for Disease Control and Prevention (CDC). (2014b). Elder abuse: Prevention and response. Retrieved from http://www.cdc.gov

11. Centers for Disease Control and Prevention (CDC). (2014c). Injury prevention and control: Division of violence prevention. Retrieved from http://www.cdc.gov

12. Centers for Disease Control and Prevention (CDC). (2015). Sexual violence definitions. Retrieved from http://www.cdc.gov

13. Child Help. (n.d.). Child abuse statistics and facts. Retrieved from https://www.childhelp.org

14. Child Welfare Information Gateway. (2013). Mandatory reporters of child

abuse and neglect. Retrieved from https://childwelfare.gov

15. Child Welfare Information Gateway. (2013). Definitions of child abuse and neglect in federal law. Retrieved from https://www.childwelfare.gov

16. Christian, C. W., Block, R., & Committee on Child Abuse and Neglect. (2009). Policy statement on abusive head trauma in infants and children. Elk Grove, IL: American Academy of Pediatrics.

17. Crane, P. (2013). Nursing interventions for human trafficking. In M. De Chesnay (Ed.), Sex Trafficking: A Clinical Guide for Nurses (pp. 167–181). New York, NY: Springer.

18. De Chesnay, M. (2013). Sex trafficking: A growing pandemic. In M. De Chesnay (Ed.), Sex Trafficking: A Clinical Guide

for Nurses (pp. 3–21). New York, NY: Springer.

19. De Chesnay, M., & Capponi, N. (2013). Emergency and community clinic policies for handling sex trafficking cases. In M. De Chesnay (Ed.), Sex Trafficking: A Clinical Guide for Nurses (pp. 295–304). New York, NY: Springer.

20. Finkelhor, D., Turner, H. A., Ormond, R., & Hamby, S. L. (2013). Updated national data on violence, crime, and abuse among children and youth. JAMA Pediatrics, 167(6), 614–621.

21. Finn, C. (2011). Forensic biomarkers in child maltreatment cases. In V. A. Lynch & J. B. Duval (Eds.), Forensic Nursing (2nd ed., pp. 341–354). St. Louis, MO: Elsevier Mosby.

22. Flaherty, E., & Resnick, B. (Eds.). (2014). Core curriculum for advanced practice

geriatric nursing. In Geriatric Nursing Review Syllabus (4th ed., pp. 97–101). New York, NY: American Geriatrics Society.

23. Futures Without Violence. (2013). Emerging issues in adolescent violence prevention. Retrieved from http://startstrong.futureswithoutviolence.org

24. International Association of Forensic Nurses. (2013). Sexual Assault Nurse Examiner (SANE) education guidelines. Elkridge, MD: International Association of Forensic Nurses.

www.ingramcontent.com/pod-product-compliance
Lightning Source LLC
Chambersburg PA
CBHW071019240526
45469CB00006BD/1985